MY 90 DAY CLEAN
&
HEALTHY EATING
JOURNAL

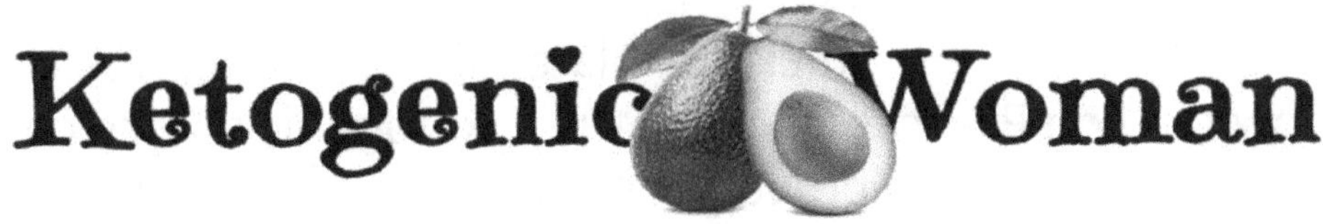

This journal was created by Anita Breeze at
www.ketogenicwoman.com

Join the conversation on Facebook at
https://www.facebook.com/groups/KetogenicWoman

Follow me on Instagram at
http://www.instagram.com/ketogenic.woman

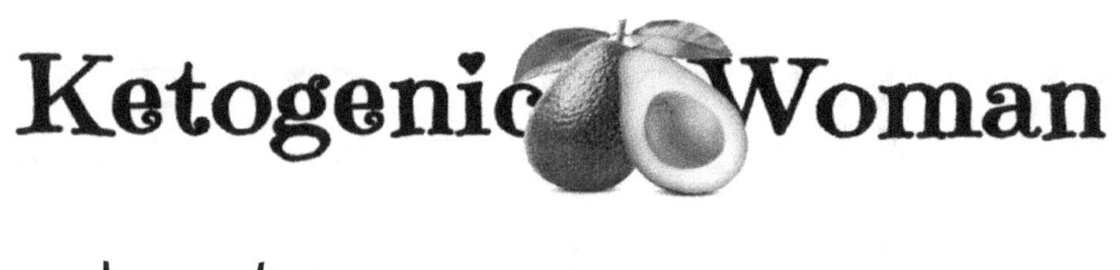

THANK YOU

As a thank you for buying my journal, I am providing you with some helpful resources that can help you along your journey.

Stuck in a plateau?
Learn how the Egg Fast can help at https://ketogenicwoman.com/egg-diet-weight-loss-fast/

Get your free printables at
https://ketogenicwoman.com/egg-fast-printables/

Get your free grocery list at
https://ketogenicwoman.com/getting-started-keto-diet-plan/

And make sure you sign up for my newsletter while you're on the site so you can get delicious recipes delivered straight to your email inbox.

Thank you for buying the My 90 Day Clean & Healthy Eating Journal!

Now, let's get started!

- Anita

DAY 1 – STARTING WEIGHT

Measurements

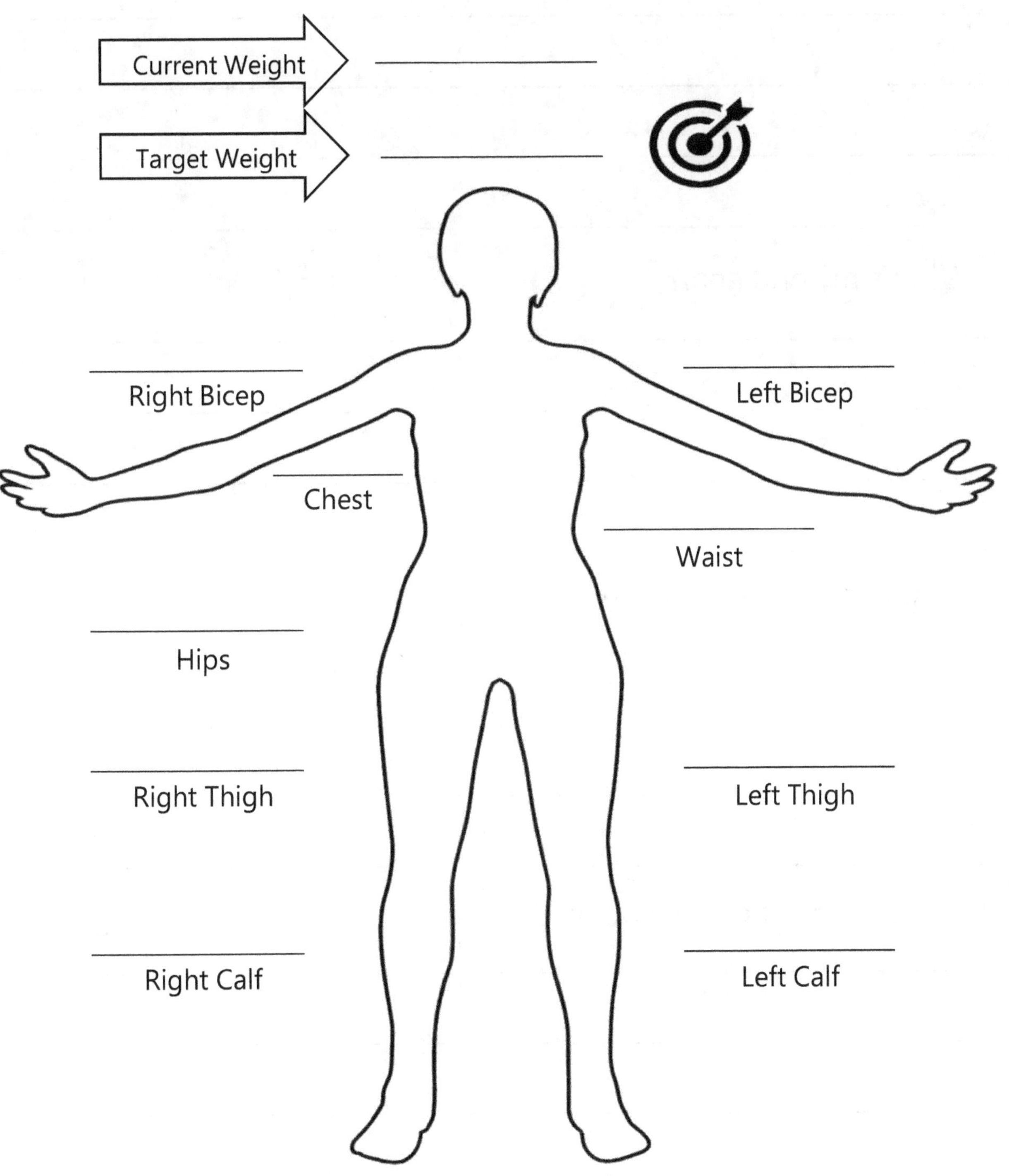

Questions To Ask Myself

Why am I starting the healthy lifestyle?

____

____

____

What's my end goal?

____

____

____

Do I have a weight loss mindset?

____

____

____

Who can I count on for support?

____

____

____

DAY 1 - 7

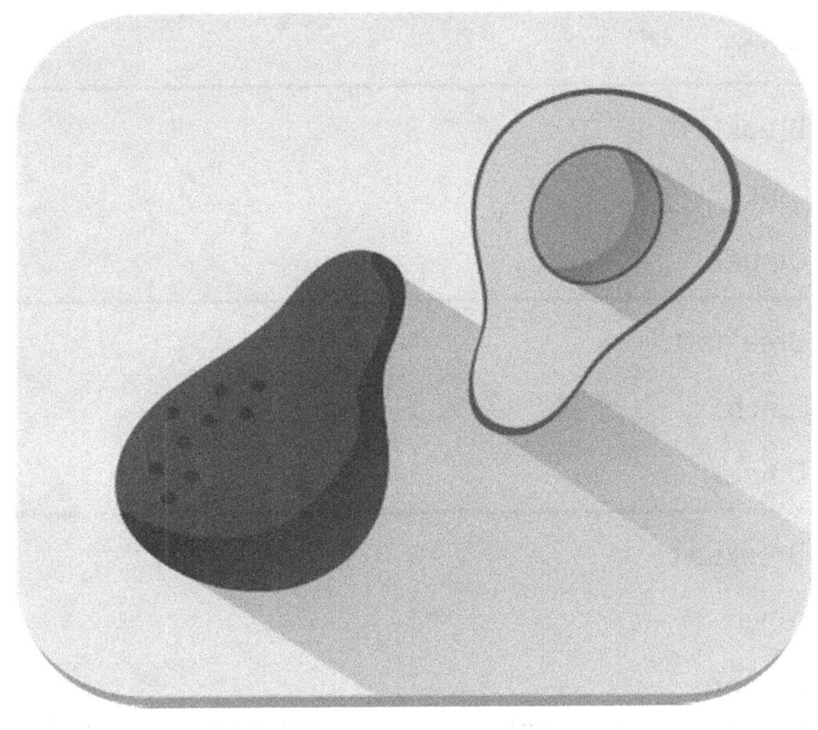

Meal Planner
Day 1 - 7

Day 1	Breakfast: Lunch: Dinner:
Day 2	Breakfast: Lunch: Dinner:
Day 3	Breakfast: Lunch: Dinner:
Day 4	Breakfast: Lunch: Dinner:
Day 5	Breakfast: Lunch: Dinner:
Day 6	Breakfast: Lunch: Dinner:
Day 7	Breakfast: Lunch: Dinner:
Snacks	

Exercise Tracker   Day 1 - 7

Day 1	Day 2	Day 3
Cardio ○ Weights ○	Cardio ○ Weights ○	Cardio ○ Weights ○

Day 4	Day 5	Day 6
Cardio ○ Weights ○	Cardio ○ Weights ○	Cardio ○ Weights ○

Day 7	Day	Calories Burned
	1	
	2	
	3	
	4	
	5	
Cardio ○	6	
Weights ○	7	

Day 1   Food Tracker

Date: _______________

MON TUE WED THU FRI SAT SUN

🎯 **Daily Target**						
Breakfast	Calories	Fat	Protein	Carbs	Fiber	Net Carbs
Total:						
Lunch	Calories	Fat	Protein	Carbs	Fiber	Net Carbs
Total:						
Dinner	Calories	Fat	Protein	Carbs	Fiber	Net Carbs
Total:						
Snacks	Calories	Fat	Protein	Carbs	Fiber	Net Carbs
Total:						
Daily Total						

Ketosis: Y/N   Intermittent Fasting: From _____am/pm - To_____am/pm

Day 2   Food Tracker

Date: ________________

MON TUE WED THU FRI SAT SUN

🎯 Daily Target						

Breakfast	Calories	Fat	Protein	Carbs	Fiber	Net Carbs
Total:						

Lunch	Calories	Fat	Protein	Carbs	Fiber	Net Carbs
Total:						

Dinner	Calories	Fat	Protein	Carbs	Fiber	Net Carbs
Total:						

Snacks	Calories	Fat	Protein	Carbs	Fiber	Net Carbs
Total:						

Daily Total						

Ketosis: Y/N   Intermittent Fasting: From ______am/pm - To______am/pm

Day 3   Food Tracker

Date: _______________

MON TUE WED THU FRI SAT SUN

🎯 **Daily Target**						

Breakfast	Calories	Fat	Protein	Carbs	Fiber	Net Carbs
Total:						

Lunch	Calories	Fat	Protein	Carbs	Fiber	Net Carbs
Total:						

Dinner	Calories	Fat	Protein	Carbs	Fiber	Net Carbs
Total:						

Snacks	Calories	Fat	Protein	Carbs	Fiber	Net Carbs
Total:						

Daily Total						

Ketosis: Y/N   Intermittent Fasting: From _______am/pm - To_______am/pm

Day 4   Food Tracker

Date: ________________
MON TUE WED THU FRI SAT SUN

⊕ **Daily Target**						
Breakfast	Calories	Fat	Protein	Carbs	Fiber	Net Carbs
Total:						
Lunch	Calories	Fat	Protein	Carbs	Fiber	Net Carbs
Total:						
Dinner	Calories	Fat	Protein	Carbs	Fiber	Net Carbs
Total:						
Snacks	Calories	Fat	Protein	Carbs	Fiber	Net Carbs
Total:						
Daily Total						

Ketosis: Y/N   Intermittent Fasting: From _____am/pm - To_____am/pm

Day 5   Food Tracker

Date: _______________

MON TUE WED THU FRI SAT SUN

⌖ Daily Target						

Breakfast	Calories	Fat	Protein	Carbs	Fiber	Net Carbs
Total:						

Lunch	Calories	Fat	Protein	Carbs	Fiber	Net Carbs
Total:						

Dinner	Calories	Fat	Protein	Carbs	Fiber	Net Carbs
Total:						

Snacks	Calories	Fat	Protein	Carbs	Fiber	Net Carbs
Total:						

Daily Total						

Ketosis: Y/N   Intermittent Fasting: From _____am/pm - To_____am/pm

Day 6   Food Tracker

Date: _______________

MON TUE WED THU FRI SAT SUN

⊕ **Daily Target**						

Breakfast	Calories	Fat	Protein	Carbs	Fiber	Net Carbs
Total:						

Lunch	Calories	Fat	Protein	Carbs	Fiber	Net Carbs
Total:						

Dinner	Calories	Fat	Protein	Carbs	Fiber	Net Carbs
Total:						

Snacks	Calories	Fat	Protein	Carbs	Fiber	Net Carbs
Total:						

Daily Total						

Ketosis: Y/N   Intermittent Fasting: From _____am/pm - To_____am/pm

Day 7　　Food Tracker

Date: ________________

MON TUE WED THU FRI SAT SUN

🎯 **Daily Target**

Breakfast	Calories	Fat	Protein	Carbs	Fiber	Net Carbs
Total:						

Lunch	Calories	Fat	Protein	Carbs	Fiber	Net Carbs
Total:						

Dinner	Calories	Fat	Protein	Carbs	Fiber	Net Carbs
Total:						

Snacks	Calories	Fat	Protein	Carbs	Fiber	Net Carbs
Total:						

| **Daily Total** | | | | | | |

Ketosis: Y/N　　Intermittent Fasting: From _____am/pm - To_____am/pm

NOTES

DAY 8 – WEIGHT

Measurements

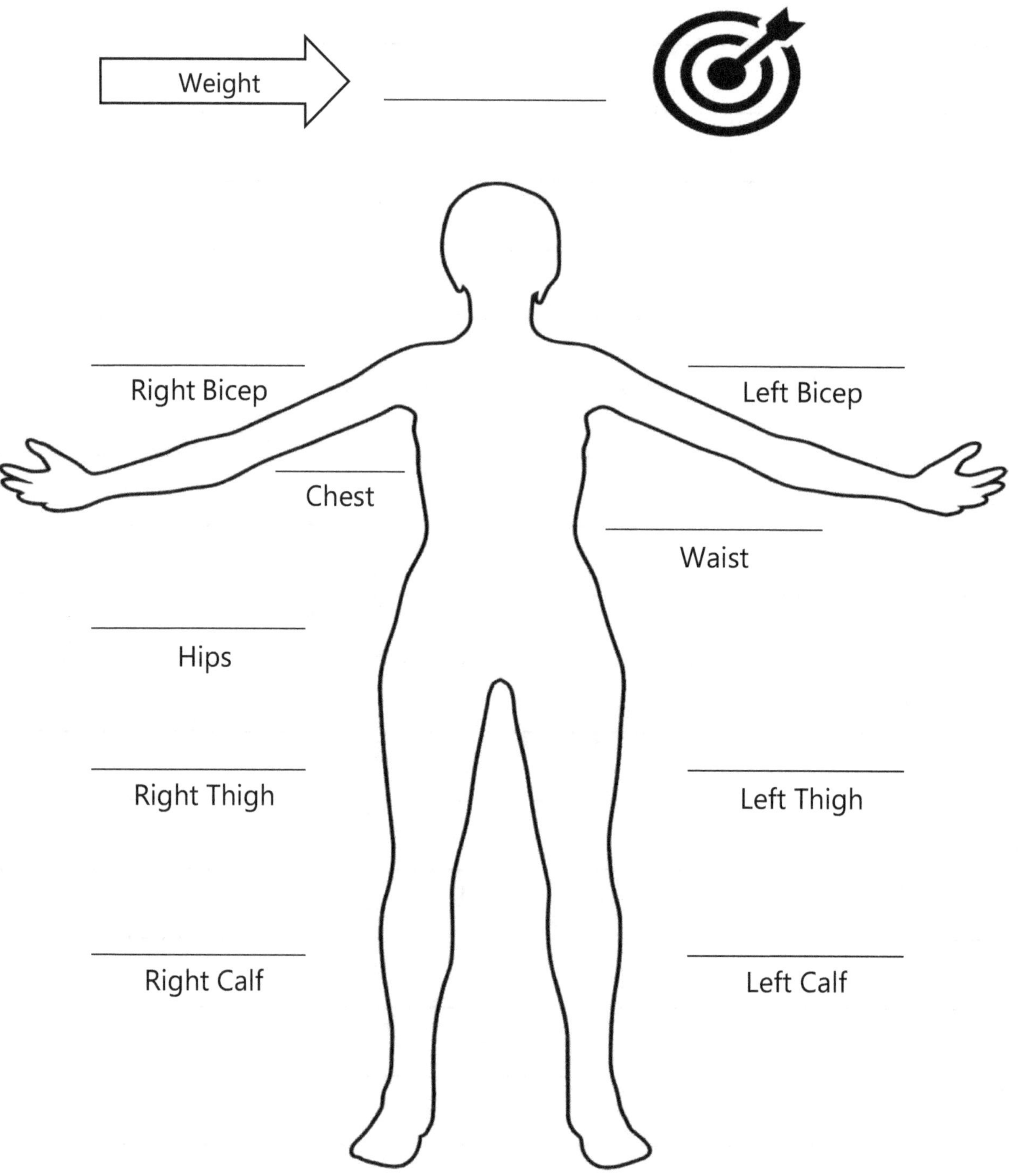

Questions To Ask Yourself

Am I happy with my results after the last 7 days?

____

____

____

____

What was my biggest win?

____

____

____

____

What adjustments should I make?

____

____

____

____

How does my body feel?

____

____

____

____

DAY 8 - 14

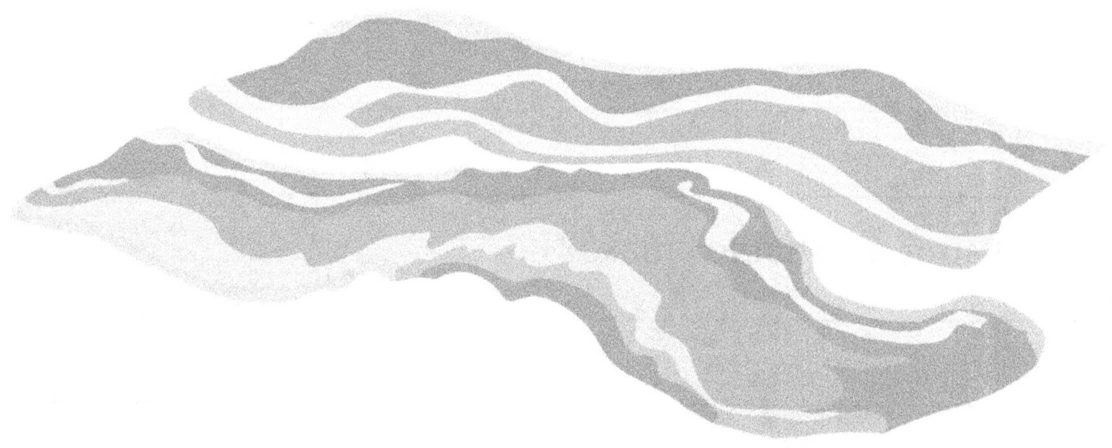

Meal Planner Day 8 - 14

Day 1	Breakfast: Lunch: Dinner:
Day 2	Breakfast: Lunch: Dinner:
Day 3	Breakfast: Lunch: Dinner:
Day 4	Breakfast: Lunch: Dinner:
Day 5	Breakfast: Lunch: Dinner:
Day 6	Breakfast: Lunch: Dinner:
Day 7	Breakfast: Lunch: Dinner:
Snacks	

Exercise Tracker

Day 8 - 14

Day 1	Day 2	Day 3
Cardio ◯ Weights ◯	Cardio ◯ Weights ◯	Cardio ◯ Weights ◯

Day 4	Day 5	Day 6
Cardio ◯ Weights ◯	Cardio ◯ Weights ◯	Cardio ◯ Weights ◯

Day 7	Day	Calories Burned
	1	
	2	
	3	
	4	
	5	
Cardio ◯	6	
Weights ◯	7	

Day 8   Food Tracker

Date: ______________

MON TUE WED THU FRI SAT SUN

🎯 **Daily Target**						

Breakfast	Calories	Fat	Protein	Carbs	Fiber	Net Carbs
Total:						

Lunch	Calories	Fat	Protein	Carbs	Fiber	Net Carbs
Total:						

Dinner	Calories	Fat	Protein	Carbs	Fiber	Net Carbs
Total:						

Snacks	Calories	Fat	Protein	Carbs	Fiber	Net Carbs
Total:						

Daily Total						

Ketosis: Y/N   Intermittent Fasting: From _____am/pm - To_____am/pm

Day 9 — Food Tracker

Date: _______________
MON TUE WED THU FRI SAT SUN

🎯 **Daily Target**						

Breakfast	Calories	Fat	Protein	Carbs	Fiber	Net Carbs
Total:						

Lunch	Calories	Fat	Protein	Carbs	Fiber	Net Carbs
Total:						

Dinner	Calories	Fat	Protein	Carbs	Fiber	Net Carbs
Total:						

Snacks	Calories	Fat	Protein	Carbs	Fiber	Net Carbs
Total:						

Daily Total						

Ketosis: Y/N   Intermittent Fasting: From _____am/pm - To_____am/pm

Day 10   Food Tracker

Date: _______________

MON TUE WED THU FRI SAT SUN

⊕ **Daily Target**						

Breakfast	Calories	Fat	Protein	Carbs	Fiber	Net Carbs
Total:						

Lunch	Calories	Fat	Protein	Carbs	Fiber	Net Carbs
Total:						

Dinner	Calories	Fat	Protein	Carbs	Fiber	Net Carbs
Total:						

Snacks	Calories	Fat	Protein	Carbs	Fiber	Net Carbs
Total:						

Daily Total						

Ketosis: Y/N   Intermittent Fasting: From _____am/pm - To_____am/pm

Day 11   Food Tracker

Date: ___________________

MON TUE WED THU FRI SAT SUN

⊕ Daily Target						

Breakfast	Calories	Fat	Protein	Carbs	Fiber	Net Carbs
Total:						

Lunch	Calories	Fat	Protein	Carbs	Fiber	Net Carbs
Total:						

Dinner	Calories	Fat	Protein	Carbs	Fiber	Net Carbs
Total:						

Snacks	Calories	Fat	Protein	Carbs	Fiber	Net Carbs
Total:						

Daily Total						

Ketosis: Y/N   Intermittent Fasting: From _____am/pm - To_____am/pm

Day 12　　Food Tracker

Date: _______________

MON TUE WED THU FRI SAT SUN

⊕ **Daily Target**						

Breakfast	Calories	Fat	Protein	Carbs	Fiber	Net Carbs
Total:						

Lunch	Calories	Fat	Protein	Carbs	Fiber	Net Carbs
Total:						

Dinner	Calories	Fat	Protein	Carbs	Fiber	Net Carbs
Total:						

Snacks	Calories	Fat	Protein	Carbs	Fiber	Net Carbs
Total:						

Daily Total						

Ketosis: Y/N　　Intermittent Fasting: From _____am/pm - To_____am/pm

Day 13   Food Tracker   Date: ___________

MON TUE WED THU FRI SAT SUN

⊕ **Daily Target**						

Breakfast	Calories	Fat	Protein	Carbs	Fiber	Net Carbs
Total:						

Lunch	Calories	Fat	Protein	Carbs	Fiber	Net Carbs
Total:						

Dinner	Calories	Fat	Protein	Carbs	Fiber	Net Carbs
Total:						

Snacks	Calories	Fat	Protein	Carbs	Fiber	Net Carbs
Total:						

Daily Total						

Ketosis: Y/N   Intermittent Fasting: From _____am/pm - To_____am/pm

Day 14   Food Tracker

Date: _______________

MON TUE WED THU FRI SAT SUN

🎯 **Daily Target**						

Breakfast	Calories	Fat	Protein	Carbs	Fiber	Net Carbs
Total:						

Lunch	Calories	Fat	Protein	Carbs	Fiber	Net Carbs
Total:						

Dinner	Calories	Fat	Protein	Carbs	Fiber	Net Carbs
Total:						

Snacks	Calories	Fat	Protein	Carbs	Fiber	Net Carbs
Total:						

Daily Total						

Ketosis: Y/N   Intermittent Fasting: From _____am/pm - To_____am/pm

NOTES

DAY 15 – WEIGHT

Measurements

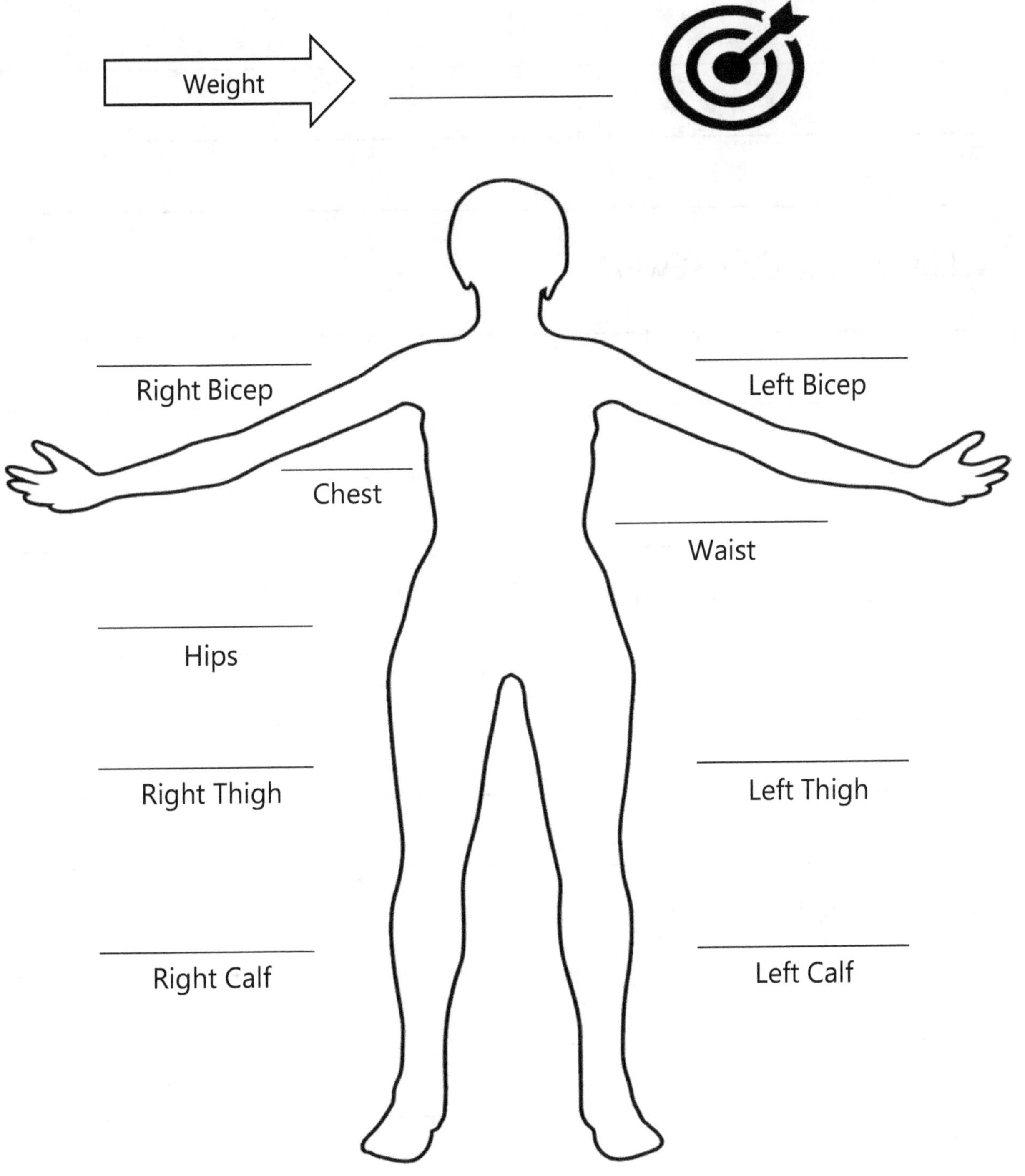

Questions To Ask Yourself

Am I happy with my results after the last 7 days?

____

____

____

____

What was my biggest win?

____

____

____

____

What adjustments should I make?

____

____

____

____

How does my body feel?

____

____

____

____

DAY 15 - 21

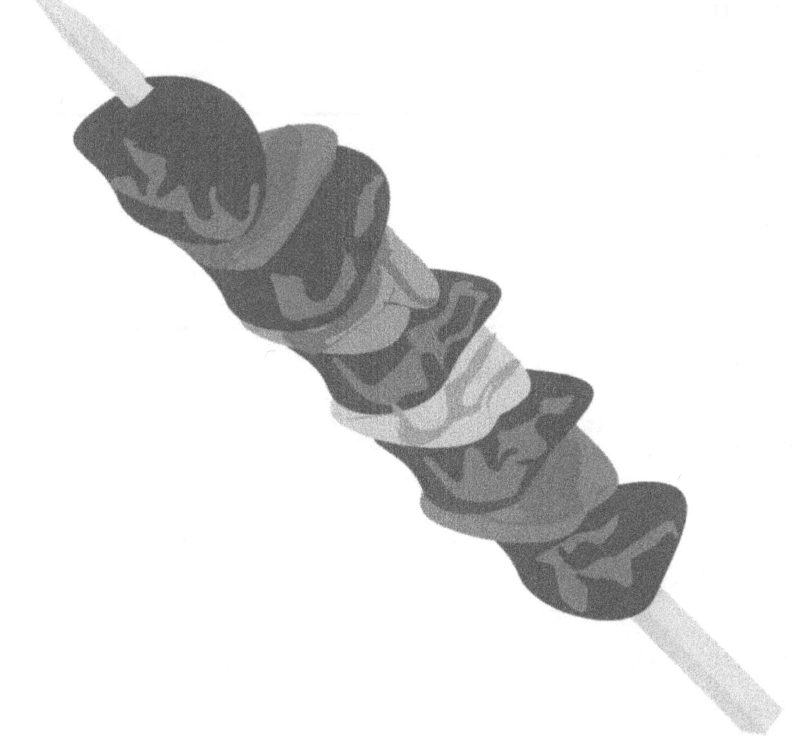

Meal Planner

Day 15 - 21

Day 1	Breakfast: Lunch: Dinner:
Day 2	Breakfast: Lunch: Dinner:
Day 3	Breakfast: Lunch: Dinner:
Day 4	Breakfast: Lunch: Dinner:
Day 5	Breakfast: Lunch: Dinner:
Day 6	Breakfast: Lunch: Dinner:
Day 7	Breakfast: Lunch: Dinner:
Snacks	

Exercise Tracker   Day 15 - 21

Day 1	Day 2	Day 3
Cardio ◯ Weights ◯	Cardio ◯ Weights ◯	Cardio ◯ Weights ◯

Day 4	Day 5	Day 6
Cardio ◯ Weights ◯	Cardio ◯ Weights ◯	Cardio ◯ Weights ◯

Day 7
Cardio ◯ Weights ◯

Day	Calories Burned
1	
2	
3	
4	
5	
6	
7	

Day 15   Food Tracker   Date: _______________

MON TUE WED THU FRI SAT SUN

⊕ **Daily Target**						
Breakfast	Calories	Fat	Protein	Carbs	Fiber	Net Carbs
Total:						
Lunch	Calories	Fat	Protein	Carbs	Fiber	Net Carbs
Total:						
Dinner	Calories	Fat	Protein	Carbs	Fiber	Net Carbs
Total:						
Snacks	Calories	Fat	Protein	Carbs	Fiber	Net Carbs
Total:						
Daily Total						

Ketosis: Y/N   Intermittent Fasting: From _____am/pm - To_____am/pm

Day 16   Food Tracker

Date: _______________

MON TUE WED THU FRI SAT SUN

🎯 **Daily Target**						

Breakfast	Calories	Fat	Protein	Carbs	Fiber	Net Carbs
Total:						

Lunch	Calories	Fat	Protein	Carbs	Fiber	Net Carbs
Total:						

Dinner	Calories	Fat	Protein	Carbs	Fiber	Net Carbs
Total:						

Snacks	Calories	Fat	Protein	Carbs	Fiber	Net Carbs
Total:						

Daily Total						

Ketosis: Y/N   Intermittent Fasting: From _____am/pm - To_____am/pm

Day 17 Food Tracker

Date: _______________

MON TUE WED THU FRI SAT SUN

⌖ **Daily Target**						

Breakfast	Calories	Fat	Protein	Carbs	Fiber	Net Carbs
Total:						

Lunch	Calories	Fat	Protein	Carbs	Fiber	Net Carbs
Total:						

Dinner	Calories	Fat	Protein	Carbs	Fiber	Net Carbs
Total:						

Snacks	Calories	Fat	Protein	Carbs	Fiber	Net Carbs
Total:						

Daily Total						

Ketosis: Y/N   Intermittent Fasting: From _____am/pm - To_____am/pm

Day 18   Food Tracker

Date: _______________

MON TUE WED THU FRI SAT SUN

⊕ Daily Target						
Breakfast	Calories	Fat	Protein	Carbs	Fiber	Net Carbs
Total:						
Lunch	Calories	Fat	Protein	Carbs	Fiber	Net Carbs
Total:						
Dinner	Calories	Fat	Protein	Carbs	Fiber	Net Carbs
Total:						
Snacks	Calories	Fat	Protein	Carbs	Fiber	Net Carbs
Total:						
Daily Total						

Ketosis: Y/N   Intermittent Fasting: From _____am/pm - To_____am/pm

Day 19   Food Tracker

Date: _______________

MON TUE WED THU FRI SAT SUN

⊕ Daily Target						

Breakfast	Calories	Fat	Protein	Carbs	Fiber	Net Carbs
Total:						

Lunch	Calories	Fat	Protein	Carbs	Fiber	Net Carbs
Total:						

Dinner	Calories	Fat	Protein	Carbs	Fiber	Net Carbs
Total:						

Snacks	Calories	Fat	Protein	Carbs	Fiber	Net Carbs
Total:						

Daily Total						

Ketosis: Y/N   Intermittent Fasting: From _____am/pm - To_____am/pm

Day 20　　Food Tracker

Date: ________________

MON TUE WED THU FRI SAT SUN

⊕ **Daily Target**						
Breakfast	Calories	Fat	Protein	Carbs	Fiber	Net Carbs
Total:						
Lunch	Calories	Fat	Protein	Carbs	Fiber	Net Carbs
Total:						
Dinner	Calories	Fat	Protein	Carbs	Fiber	Net Carbs
Total:						
Snacks	Calories	Fat	Protein	Carbs	Fiber	Net Carbs
Total:						
Daily Total						

Ketosis: Y/N　　Intermittent Fasting: From _____am/pm - To_____am/pm

Day 21   Food Tracker

Date: ___________________

MON TUE WED THU FRI SAT SUN

🎯 Daily Target						

Breakfast	Calories	Fat	Protein	Carbs	Fiber	Net Carbs
Total:						

Lunch	Calories	Fat	Protein	Carbs	Fiber	Net Carbs
Total:						

Dinner	Calories	Fat	Protein	Carbs	Fiber	Net Carbs
Total:						

Snacks	Calories	Fat	Protein	Carbs	Fiber	Net Carbs
Total:						

Daily Total						

Ketosis: Y/N   Intermittent Fasting: From ______am/pm - To______am/pm

NOTES

DAY 22 – WEIGHT

Measurements

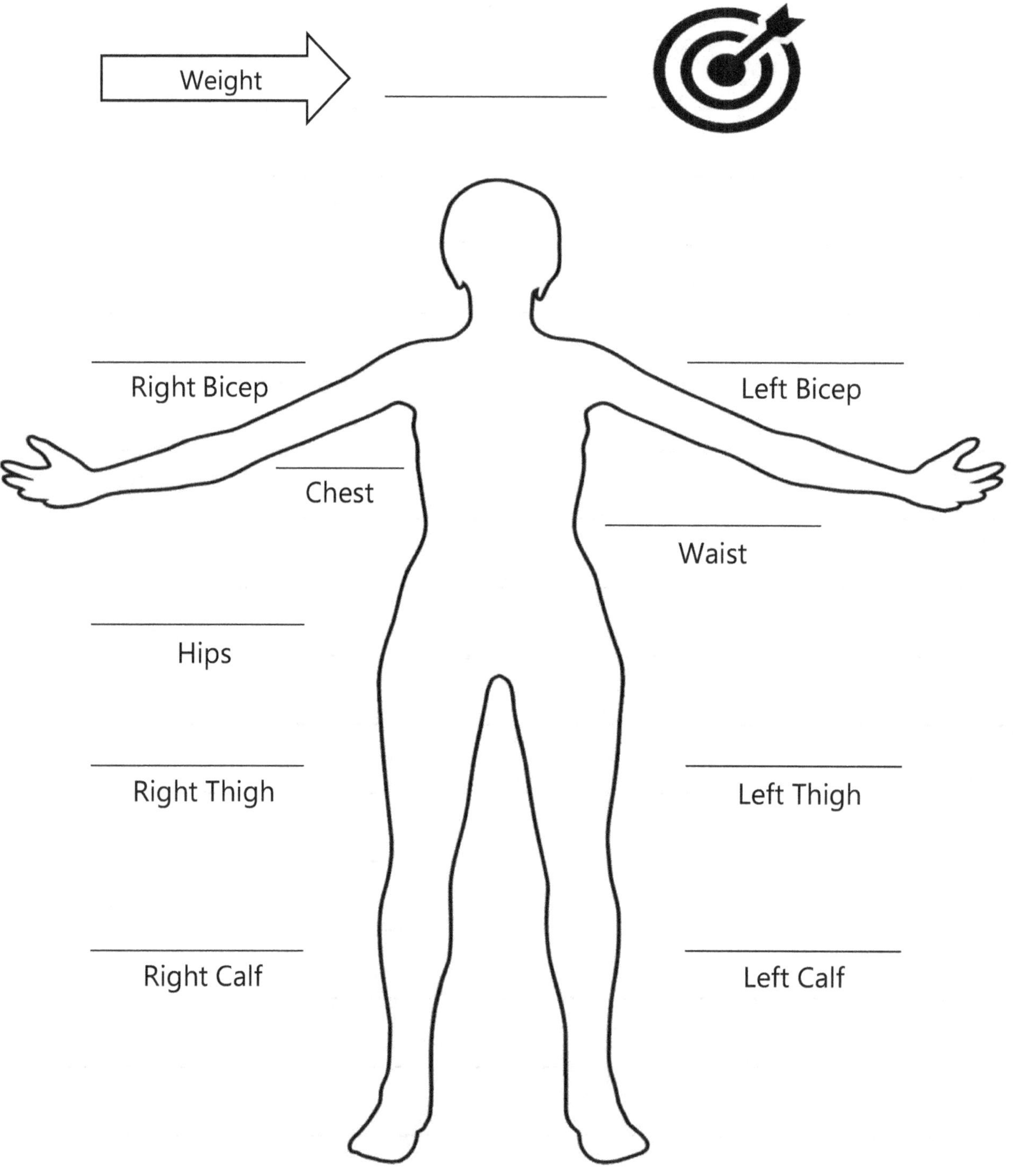

Questions To Ask Yourself

Am I happy with my results after the last 7 days?

____

____

____

____

What was my biggest win?

____

____

____

____

What adjustments should I make?

____

____

____

____

How does my body feel?

____

____

____

____

DAY 22 - 28

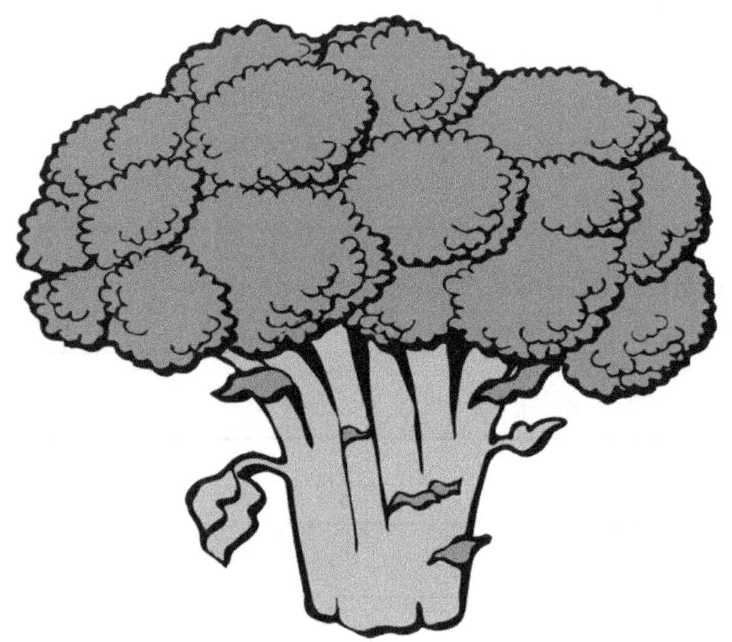

Meal Planner   Day 22 - 28

Day 1	Breakfast: Lunch: Dinner:
Day 2	Breakfast: Lunch: Dinner:
Day 3	Breakfast: Lunch: Dinner:
Day 4	Breakfast: Lunch: Dinner:
Day 5	Breakfast: Lunch: Dinner:
Day 6	Breakfast: Lunch: Dinner:
Day 7	Breakfast: Lunch: Dinner:
Snacks	

Exercise Tracker

Day 22 - 28

Day 1

Cardio ○
Weights ○

Day 2

Cardio ○
Weights ○

Day 3

Cardio ○
Weights ○

Day 4

Cardio ○
Weights ○

Day 5

Cardio ○
Weights ○

Day 6

Cardio ○
Weights ○

Day 7

Cardio ○
Weights ○

Day	Calories Burned
1	
2	
3	
4	
5	
6	
7	

Day 22   Food Tracker

Date: _______________

MON TUE WED THU FRI SAT SUN

🎯 **Daily Target**						
Breakfast	Calories	Fat	Protein	Carbs	Fiber	Net Carbs
Total:						
Lunch	Calories	Fat	Protein	Carbs	Fiber	Net Carbs
Total:						
Dinner	Calories	Fat	Protein	Carbs	Fiber	Net Carbs
Total:						
Snacks	Calories	Fat	Protein	Carbs	Fiber	Net Carbs
Total:						
Daily Total						

Ketosis: Y/N   Intermittent Fasting: From _____am/pm - To_____am/pm

Day 23 Food Tracker

Date: _______________

MON TUE WED THU FRI SAT SUN

⊕ Daily Target						

Breakfast	Calories	Fat	Protein	Carbs	Fiber	Net Carbs
Total:						

Lunch	Calories	Fat	Protein	Carbs	Fiber	Net Carbs
Total:						

Dinner	Calories	Fat	Protein	Carbs	Fiber	Net Carbs
Total:						

Snacks	Calories	Fat	Protein	Carbs	Fiber	Net Carbs
Total:						

Daily Total						

Ketosis: Y/N   Intermittent Fasting: From _____am/pm - To_____am/pm

Day 24   Food Tracker

Date: _______________

MON TUE WED THU FRI SAT SUN

⌖ Daily Target						

Breakfast	Calories	Fat	Protein	Carbs	Fiber	Net Carbs
Total:						

Lunch	Calories	Fat	Protein	Carbs	Fiber	Net Carbs
Total:						

Dinner	Calories	Fat	Protein	Carbs	Fiber	Net Carbs
Total:						

Snacks	Calories	Fat	Protein	Carbs	Fiber	Net Carbs
Total:						

Daily Total						

Ketosis: Y/N   Intermittent Fasting: From _____am/pm - To_____am/pm

Day 25   Food Tracker

Date: _______________

MON TUE WED THU FRI SAT SUN

⌖ **Daily Target**						

Breakfast	Calories	Fat	Protein	Carbs	Fiber	Net Carbs
Total:						

Lunch	Calories	Fat	Protein	Carbs	Fiber	Net Carbs
Total:						

Dinner	Calories	Fat	Protein	Carbs	Fiber	Net Carbs
Total:						

Snacks	Calories	Fat	Protein	Carbs	Fiber	Net Carbs
Total:						

Daily Total						

Ketosis: Y/N   Intermittent Fasting: From _____am/pm - To_____am/pm

Day 26　　Food Tracker

Date: _______________
MON TUE WED THU FRI SAT SUN

⊕ Daily Target						

Breakfast	Calories	Fat	Protein	Carbs	Fiber	Net Carbs
Total:						

Lunch	Calories	Fat	Protein	Carbs	Fiber	Net Carbs
Total:						

Dinner	Calories	Fat	Protein	Carbs	Fiber	Net Carbs
Total:						

Snacks	Calories	Fat	Protein	Carbs	Fiber	Net Carbs
Total:						

Daily Total						

Ketosis:　Y/N　Intermittent Fasting: From _____am/pm - To_____am/pm

Day 27   Food Tracker

Date: ________________

MON TUE WED THU FRI SAT SUN

⊕ **Daily Target**						

Breakfast	Calories	Fat	Protein	Carbs	Fiber	Net Carbs
Total:						

Lunch	Calories	Fat	Protein	Carbs	Fiber	Net Carbs
Total:						

Dinner	Calories	Fat	Protein	Carbs	Fiber	Net Carbs
Total:						

Snacks	Calories	Fat	Protein	Carbs	Fiber	Net Carbs
Total:						

Daily Total						

Ketosis: Y/N   Intermittent Fasting: From _____am/pm - To_____am/pm

Day 28   Food Tracker

Date: ________________

MON TUE WED THU FRI SAT SUN

⊕ **Daily Target**

Breakfast	Calories	Fat	Protein	Carbs	Fiber	Net Carbs
Total:						

Lunch	Calories	Fat	Protein	Carbs	Fiber	Net Carbs
Total:						

Dinner	Calories	Fat	Protein	Carbs	Fiber	Net Carbs
Total:						

Snacks	Calories	Fat	Protein	Carbs	Fiber	Net Carbs
Total:						
Daily Total						

Ketosis: Y/N   Intermittent Fasting: From _____am/pm - To_____am/pm

NOTES

DAY 29 – WEIGHT

Measurements

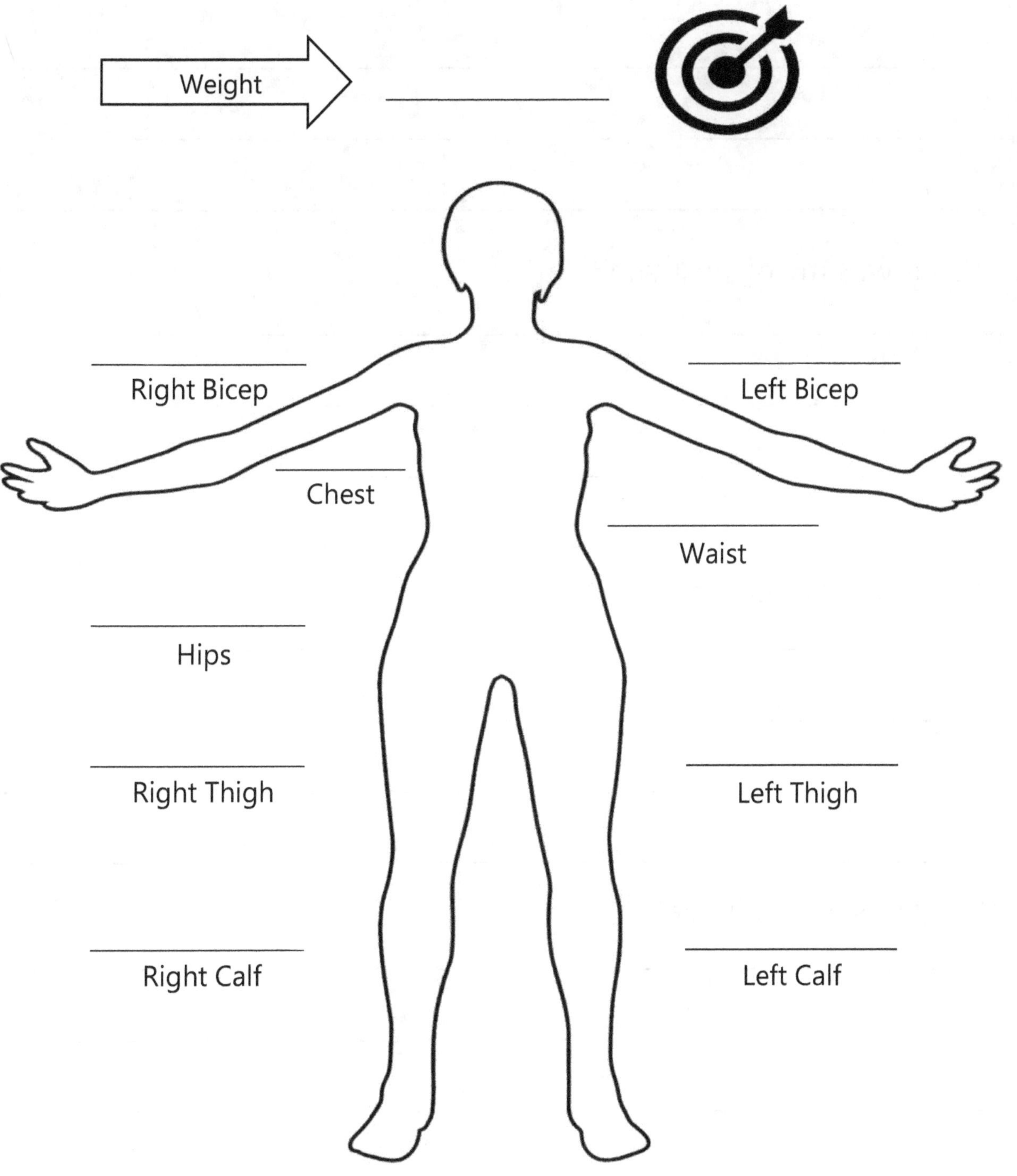

Questions To Ask Yourself

Am I happy with my results after the last 7 days?

What was my biggest win?

What adjustments should I make?

How does my body feel?

DAY 29 - 35

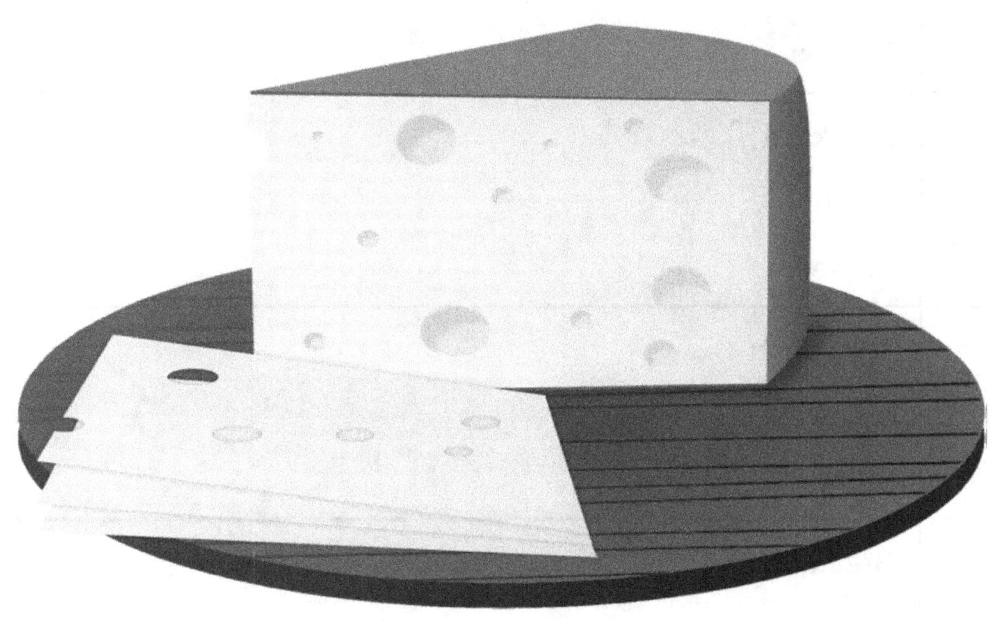

Meal Planner

Day 1	Breakfast: Lunch: Dinner:
Day 2	Breakfast: Lunch: Dinner:
Day 3	Breakfast: Lunch: Dinner:
Day 4	Breakfast: Lunch: Dinner:
Day 5	Breakfast: Lunch: Dinner:
Day 6	Breakfast: Lunch: Dinner:
Day 7	Breakfast: Lunch: Dinner:
Snacks	

Exercise Tracker

Day 1	Day 2	Day 3
Cardio ◯ Weights ◯	Cardio ◯ Weights ◯	Cardio ◯ Weights ◯

Day 4	Day 5	Day 6
Cardio ◯ Weights ◯	Cardio ◯ Weights ◯	Cardio ◯ Weights ◯

Day 7
Cardio ◯ Weights ◯

Day	Calories Burned
1	
2	
3	
4	
5	
6	
7	

Day 29   Food Tracker

Date: _________________________

MON TUE WED THU FRI SAT SUN

⊕ **Daily Target**

Breakfast	Calories	Fat	Protein	Carbs	Fiber	Net Carbs
Total:						

Lunch	Calories	Fat	Protein	Carbs	Fiber	Net Carbs
Total:						

Dinner	Calories	Fat	Protein	Carbs	Fiber	Net Carbs
Total:						

Snacks	Calories	Fat	Protein	Carbs	Fiber	Net Carbs
Total:						

| **Daily Total** | | | | | | |

Ketosis: Y/N   Intermittent Fasting: From ______am/pm - To______am/pm

Day 30   Food Tracker

Date: ________________

MON TUE WED THU FRI SAT SUN

⊕ Daily Target						
Breakfast	Calories	Fat	Protein	Carbs	Fiber	Net Carbs
Total:						
Lunch	Calories	Fat	Protein	Carbs	Fiber	Net Carbs
Total:						
Dinner	Calories	Fat	Protein	Carbs	Fiber	Net Carbs
Total:						
Snacks	Calories	Fat	Protein	Carbs	Fiber	Net Carbs
Total:						
Daily Total						

Ketosis: Y/N   Intermittent Fasting: From _____am/pm - To_____am/pm

Day 31   Food Tracker

Date: ___________

MON TUE WED THU FRI SAT SUN

⊕ Daily Target						
Breakfast	Calories	Fat	Protein	Carbs	Fiber	Net Carbs
Total:						
Lunch	Calories	Fat	Protein	Carbs	Fiber	Net Carbs
Total:						
Dinner	Calories	Fat	Protein	Carbs	Fiber	Net Carbs
Total:						
Snacks	Calories	Fat	Protein	Carbs	Fiber	Net Carbs
Total:						
Daily Total						

Ketosis: Y/N   Intermittent Fasting: From _____am/pm - To_____am/pm

Day 32   Food Tracker

Date: _______________

MON TUE WED THU FRI SAT SUN

🎯 Daily Target						

Breakfast	Calories	Fat	Protein	Carbs	Fiber	Net Carbs
Total:						

Lunch	Calories	Fat	Protein	Carbs	Fiber	Net Carbs
Total:						

Dinner	Calories	Fat	Protein	Carbs	Fiber	Net Carbs
Total:						

Snacks	Calories	Fat	Protein	Carbs	Fiber	Net Carbs
Total:						

Daily Total						

Ketosis: Y/N   Intermittent Fasting: From _____am/pm - To_____am/pm

Day 33   Food Tracker

Date: _______________
MON TUE WED THU FRI SAT SUN

Daily Target

Breakfast	Calories	Fat	Protein	Carbs	Fiber	Net Carbs
Total:						

Lunch	Calories	Fat	Protein	Carbs	Fiber	Net Carbs
Total:						

Dinner	Calories	Fat	Protein	Carbs	Fiber	Net Carbs
Total:						

Snacks	Calories	Fat	Protein	Carbs	Fiber	Net Carbs
Total:						

| **Daily Total** | | | | | | |

Ketosis: Y/N   Intermittent Fasting: From _____am/pm - To_____am/pm

Day 34   Food Tracker

Date: _______________

MON TUE WED THU FRI SAT SUN

⊕ Daily Target						

Breakfast	Calories	Fat	Protein	Carbs	Fiber	Net Carbs
Total:						

Lunch	Calories	Fat	Protein	Carbs	Fiber	Net Carbs
Total:						

Dinner	Calories	Fat	Protein	Carbs	Fiber	Net Carbs
Total:						

Snacks	Calories	Fat	Protein	Carbs	Fiber	Net Carbs
Daily Total						

Ketosis: Y/N   Intermittent Fasting: From _____am/pm - To_____am/pm

Day 35   Food Tracker

Date: _______________

MON TUE WED THU FRI SAT SUN

⊕ **Daily Target**						

Breakfast	Calories	Fat	Protein	Carbs	Fiber	Net Carbs
Total:						

Lunch	Calories	Fat	Protein	Carbs	Fiber	Net Carbs
Total:						

Dinner	Calories	Fat	Protein	Carbs	Fiber	Net Carbs
Total:						

Snacks	Calories	Fat	Protein	Carbs	Fiber	Net Carbs
Total:						

Daily Total						

Ketosis: Y/N   Intermittent Fasting: From _____am/pm - To_____am/pm

NOTES

DAY 36 – WEIGHT

Measurements

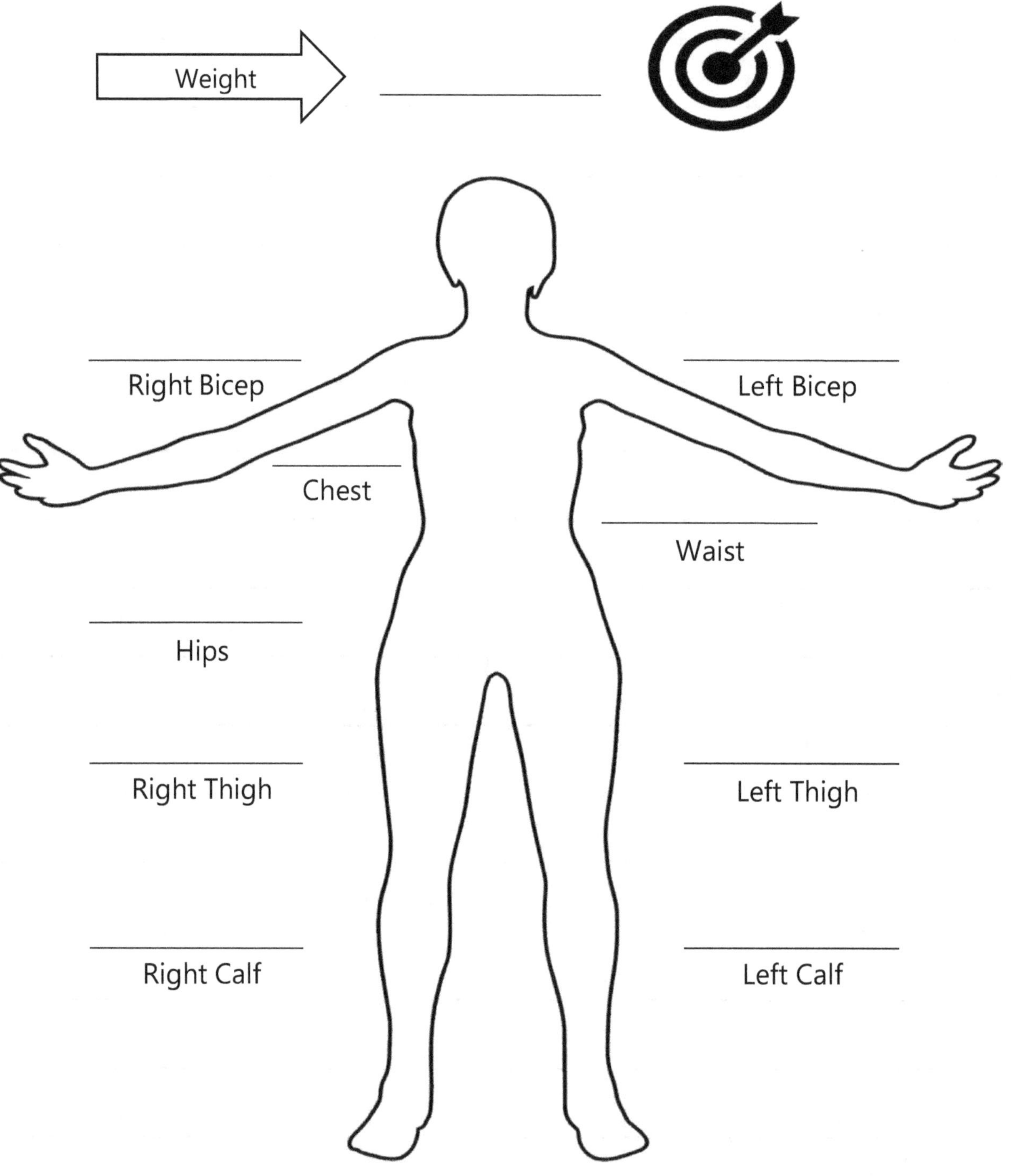

Questions To Ask Yourself

Am I happy with my results after the last 7 days?

____

____

____

____

What was my biggest win?

____

____

____

____

What adjustments should I make?

____

____

____

How does my body feel?

____

____

____

____

DAY 36 - 42

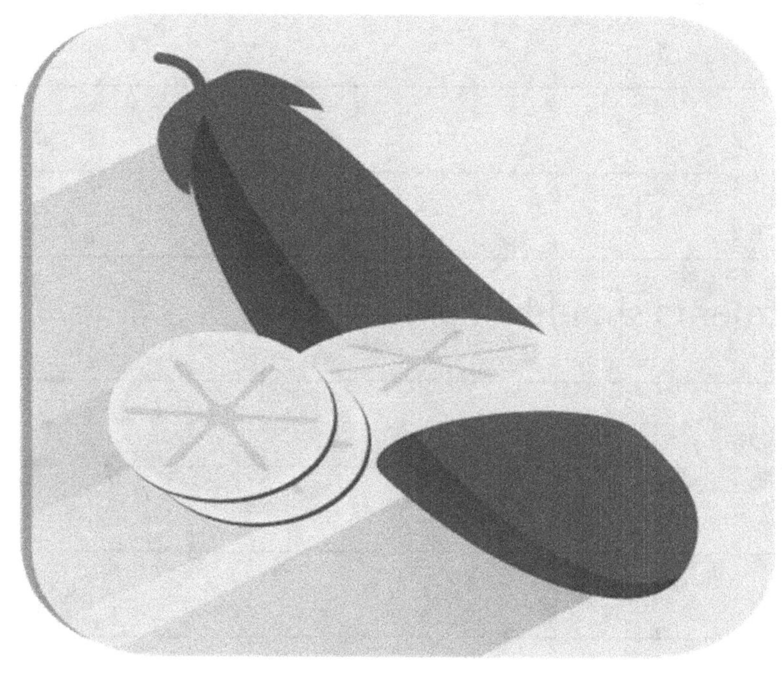

Meal Planner Day 36 - 42

Day 1	Breakfast: Lunch: Dinner:
Day 2	Breakfast: Lunch: Dinner:
Day 3	Breakfast: Lunch: Dinner:
Day 4	Breakfast: Lunch: Dinner:
Day 5	Breakfast: Lunch: Dinner:
Day 6	Breakfast: Lunch: Dinner:
Day 7	Breakfast: Lunch: Dinner:
Snacks	

Exercise Tracker   Day 36 - 42

Day 1

Cardio ⭘
Weights ⭘

Day 2

Cardio ⭘
Weights ⭘

Day 3

Cardio ⭘
Weights ⭘

Day 4

Cardio ⭘
Weights ⭘

Day 5

Cardio ⭘
Weights ⭘

Day 6

Cardio ⭘
Weights ⭘

Day 7

Cardio ⭘
Weights ⭘

Day	Calories Burned
1	
2	
3	
4	
5	
6	
7	

Day 36   Food Tracker

Date: ________________

MON TUE WED THU FRI SAT SUN

🎯 Daily Target						

Breakfast	Calories	Fat	Protein	Carbs	Fiber	Net Carbs
Total:						

Lunch	Calories	Fat	Protein	Carbs	Fiber	Net Carbs
Total:						

Dinner	Calories	Fat	Protein	Carbs	Fiber	Net Carbs
Total:						

Snacks	Calories	Fat	Protein	Carbs	Fiber	Net Carbs
Total:						

Daily Total						

Ketosis: Y/N   Intermittent Fasting: From _____am/pm - To_____am/pm

Day 37   Food Tracker

Date: _______________

MON TUE WED THU FRI SAT SUN

⊕ **Daily Target**

Breakfast	Calories	Fat	Protein	Carbs	Fiber	Net Carbs
Total:						

Lunch	Calories	Fat	Protein	Carbs	Fiber	Net Carbs
Total:						

Dinner	Calories	Fat	Protein	Carbs	Fiber	Net Carbs
Total:						

Snacks	Calories	Fat	Protein	Carbs	Fiber	Net Carbs
Total:						

| **Daily Total** | | | | | | |

Ketosis: Y/N   Intermittent Fasting: From _____am/pm - To_____am/pm

Day 38   Food Tracker

Date: _______________

MON TUE WED THU FRI SAT SUN

Daily Target

Breakfast	Calories	Fat	Protein	Carbs	Fiber	Net Carbs
Total:						

Lunch	Calories	Fat	Protein	Carbs	Fiber	Net Carbs
Total:						

Dinner	Calories	Fat	Protein	Carbs	Fiber	Net Carbs
Total:						

Snacks	Calories	Fat	Protein	Carbs	Fiber	Net Carbs
Total:						

| **Daily Total** | | | | | | |

Ketosis: Y/N   Intermittent Fasting: From _____am/pm - To_____am/pm

Day 39　Food Tracker

Date: _______________

MON TUE WED THU FRI SAT SUN

⊕ **Daily Target**

Breakfast	Calories	Fat	Protein	Carbs	Fiber	Net Carbs
Total:						

Lunch	Calories	Fat	Protein	Carbs	Fiber	Net Carbs
Total:						

Dinner	Calories	Fat	Protein	Carbs	Fiber	Net Carbs
Total:						

Snacks	Calories	Fat	Protein	Carbs	Fiber	Net Carbs
Total:						

| **Daily Total** | | | | | | |

Ketosis: Y/N　Intermittent Fasting: From _____am/pm - To_____am/pm

Day 40   Food Tracker

Date: _______________

MON TUE WED THU FRI SAT SUN

⌖ **Daily Target**						
Breakfast	Calories	Fat	Protein	Carbs	Fiber	Net Carbs
Total:						
Lunch	Calories	Fat	Protein	Carbs	Fiber	Net Carbs
Total:						
Dinner	Calories	Fat	Protein	Carbs	Fiber	Net Carbs
Total:						
Snacks	Calories	Fat	Protein	Carbs	Fiber	Net Carbs
Total:						
Daily Total						

Ketosis: Y/N   Intermittent Fasting: From _____am/pm - To_____am/pm

Day 41   Food Tracker   Date: ___________

MON TUE WED THU FRI SAT SUN

⊕ **Daily Target**

Breakfast	Calories	Fat	Protein	Carbs	Fiber	Net Carbs
Total:						

Lunch	Calories	Fat	Protein	Carbs	Fiber	Net Carbs
Total:						

Dinner	Calories	Fat	Protein	Carbs	Fiber	Net Carbs
Total:						

Snacks	Calories	Fat	Protein	Carbs	Fiber	Net Carbs
Total:						

| **Daily Total** | | | | | | |

Ketosis: Y/N   Intermittent Fasting: From _____am/pm - To_____am/pm

Day 42 Food Tracker

Date: _______________
MON TUE WED THU FRI SAT SUN

⊕ **Daily Target**						
Breakfast	Calories	Fat	Protein	Carbs	Fiber	Net Carbs
Total:						
Lunch	Calories	Fat	Protein	Carbs	Fiber	Net Carbs
Total:						
Dinner	Calories	Fat	Protein	Carbs	Fiber	Net Carbs
Total:						
Snacks	Calories	Fat	Protein	Carbs	Fiber	Net Carbs
Total:						
Daily Total						

Ketosis: Y/N   Intermittent Fasting: From _____am/pm - To_____am/pm

NOTES

DAY 43 – WEIGHT

Measurements

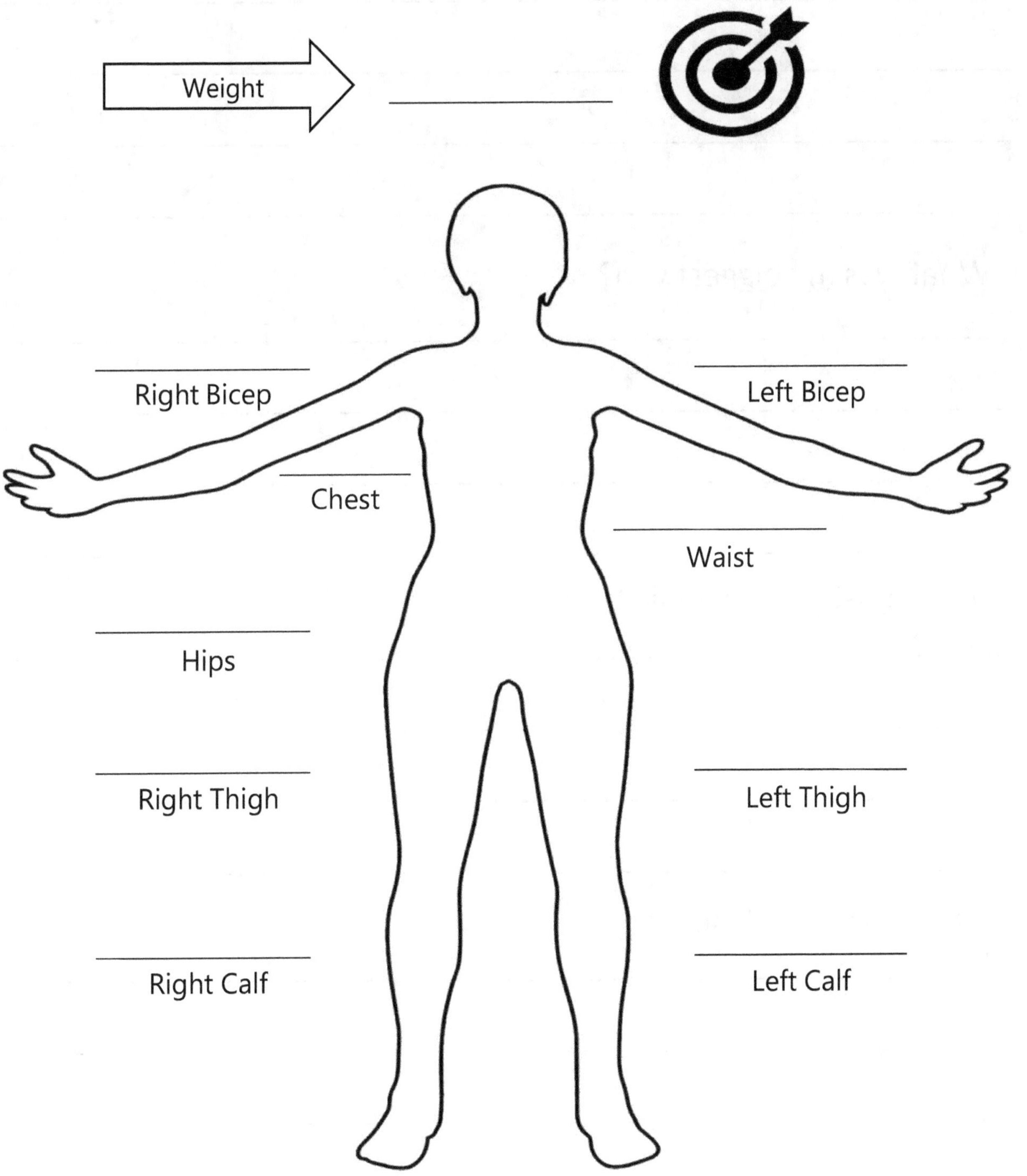

Questions To Ask Yourself

Am I happy with my results after the last 7 days?

____

____

____

What was my biggest win?

____

____

____

What adjustments should I make?

____

____

____

How does my body feel?

____

____

____

DAY 43 - 49

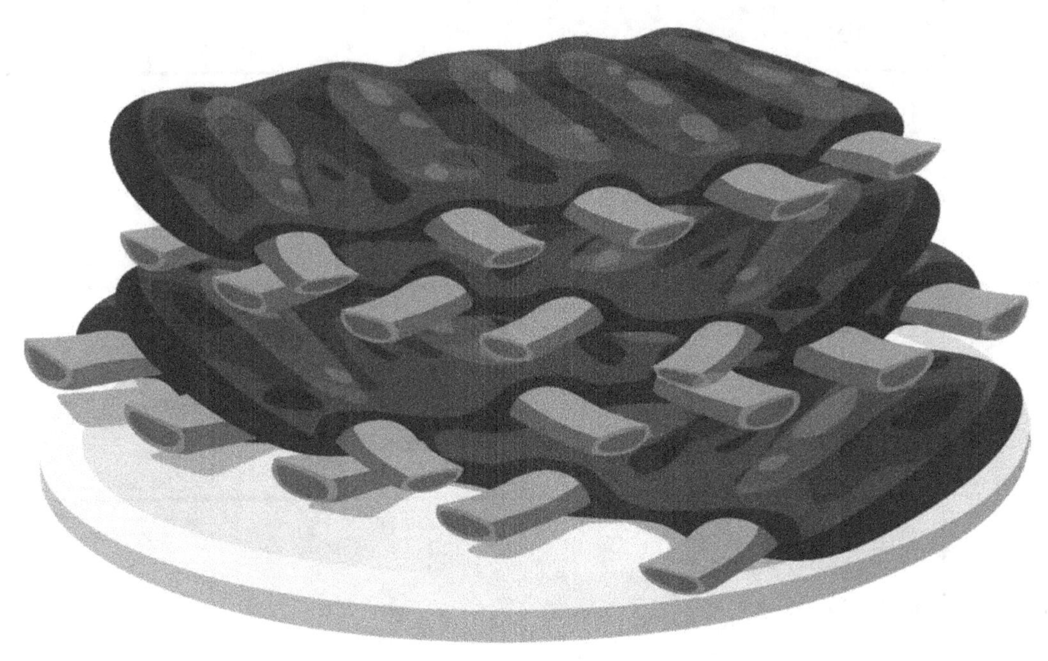

Meal Planner   Day 43 - 49

Day 1	Breakfast: Lunch: Dinner:
Day 2	Breakfast: Lunch: Dinner:
Day 3	Breakfast: Lunch: Dinner:
Day 4	Breakfast: Lunch: Dinner:
Day 5	Breakfast: Lunch: Dinner:
Day 6	Breakfast: Lunch: Dinner:
Day 7	Breakfast: Lunch: Dinner:
Snacks	

Exercise Tracker   Day 43 - 49

Day 1	Day 2	Day 3
Cardio ◯ Weights ◯	Cardio ◯ Weights ◯	Cardio ◯ Weights ◯

Day 4	Day 5	Day 6
Cardio ◯ Weights ◯	Cardio ◯ Weights ◯	Cardio ◯ Weights ◯

Day 7		Day	Calories Burned
		1	
		2	
		3	
		4	
		5	
Cardio ◯		6	
Weights ◯		7	

Day 43　　Food Tracker

Date: ________________

MON TUE WED THU FRI SAT SUN

⊕ **Daily Target**

Breakfast	Calories	Fat	Protein	Carbs	Fiber	Net Carbs
Total:						

Lunch	Calories	Fat	Protein	Carbs	Fiber	Net Carbs
Total:						

Dinner	Calories	Fat	Protein	Carbs	Fiber	Net Carbs
Total:						

Snacks	Calories	Fat	Protein	Carbs	Fiber	Net Carbs
Total:						

Daily Total						

Ketosis:　Y/N　　Intermittent Fasting: From _____am/pm - To_____am/pm

Day 44 Food Tracker

Date: _______________

MON TUE WED THU FRI SAT SUN

⊕ Daily Target					

Breakfast	Calories	Fat	Protein	Carbs	Fiber	Net Carbs
Total:						

Lunch	Calories	Fat	Protein	Carbs	Fiber	Net Carbs
Total:						

Dinner	Calories	Fat	Protein	Carbs	Fiber	Net Carbs
Total:						

Snacks	Calories	Fat	Protein	Carbs	Fiber	Net Carbs
Total:						

Daily Total					

Ketosis: Y/N   Intermittent Fasting: From _____am/pm - To_____am/pm

Day 45   Food Tracker

Date: ___________________
MON TUE WED THU FRI SAT SUN

⊕ Daily Target						
Breakfast	Calories	Fat	Protein	Carbs	Fiber	Net Carbs
Total:						
Lunch	Calories	Fat	Protein	Carbs	Fiber	Net Carbs
Total:						
Dinner	Calories	Fat	Protein	Carbs	Fiber	Net Carbs
Total:						
Snacks	Calories	Fat	Protein	Carbs	Fiber	Net Carbs
Total:						
Daily Total						

Ketosis: Y/N   Intermittent Fasting: From _____am/pm - To_____am/pm

Day 46   Food Tracker

Date: __________________

MON TUE WED THU FRI SAT SUN

🎯 **Daily Target**						

Breakfast	Calories	Fat	Protein	Carbs	Fiber	Net Carbs
Total:						

Lunch	Calories	Fat	Protein	Carbs	Fiber	Net Carbs
Total:						

Dinner	Calories	Fat	Protein	Carbs	Fiber	Net Carbs
Total:						

Snacks	Calories	Fat	Protein	Carbs	Fiber	Net Carbs
Total:						

Daily Total						

Ketosis: Y/N   Intermittent Fasting: From _____am/pm - To_____am/pm

Day 47   Food Tracker

Date: _______________

MON TUE WED THU FRI SAT SUN

⌖ Daily Target						
Breakfast	Calories	Fat	Protein	Carbs	Fiber	Net Carbs
Total:						
Lunch	Calories	Fat	Protein	Carbs	Fiber	Net Carbs
Total:						
Dinner	Calories	Fat	Protein	Carbs	Fiber	Net Carbs
Total:						
Snacks	Calories	Fat	Protein	Carbs	Fiber	Net Carbs
Total:						
Daily Total						

Ketosis: Y/N   Intermittent Fasting: From _____am/pm - To_____am/pm

Day 48   Food Tracker

Date: _______________________

MON TUE WED THU FRI SAT SUN

⊕ Daily Target

Breakfast	Calories	Fat	Protein	Carbs	Fiber	Net Carbs
Total:						

Lunch	Calories	Fat	Protein	Carbs	Fiber	Net Carbs
Total:						

Dinner	Calories	Fat	Protein	Carbs	Fiber	Net Carbs
Total:						

Snacks	Calories	Fat	Protein	Carbs	Fiber	Net Carbs
Total:						

| **Daily Total** | | | | | | |

Ketosis: Y/N   Intermittent Fasting: From _____am/pm - To_____am/pm

Day 49   Food Tracker

Date: ____________________

MON TUE WED THU FRI SAT SUN

⊕ **Daily Target**						

Breakfast	Calories	Fat	Protein	Carbs	Fiber	Net Carbs
Total:						

Lunch	Calories	Fat	Protein	Carbs	Fiber	Net Carbs
Total:						

Dinner	Calories	Fat	Protein	Carbs	Fiber	Net Carbs
Total:						

Snacks	Calories	Fat	Protein	Carbs	Fiber	Net Carbs
Total:						

Daily Total						

Ketosis: Y/N   Intermittent Fasting: From _____am/pm - To_____am/pm

NOTES

DAY 50 – WEIGHT

Measurements

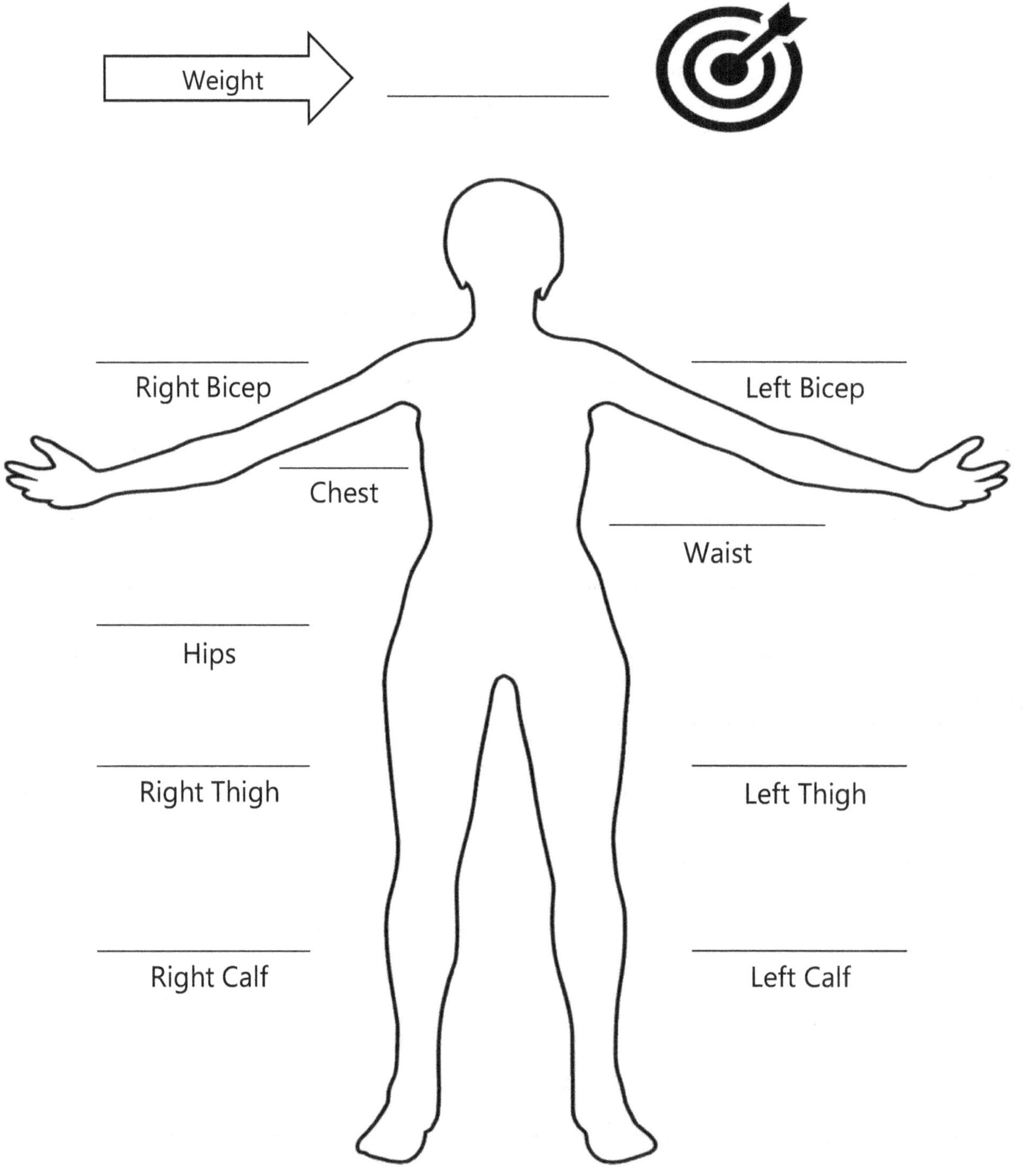

Questions To Ask Yourself

Am I happy with my results after the last 7 days?

What was my biggest win?

What adjustments should I make?

How does my body feel?

DAY 50 - 56

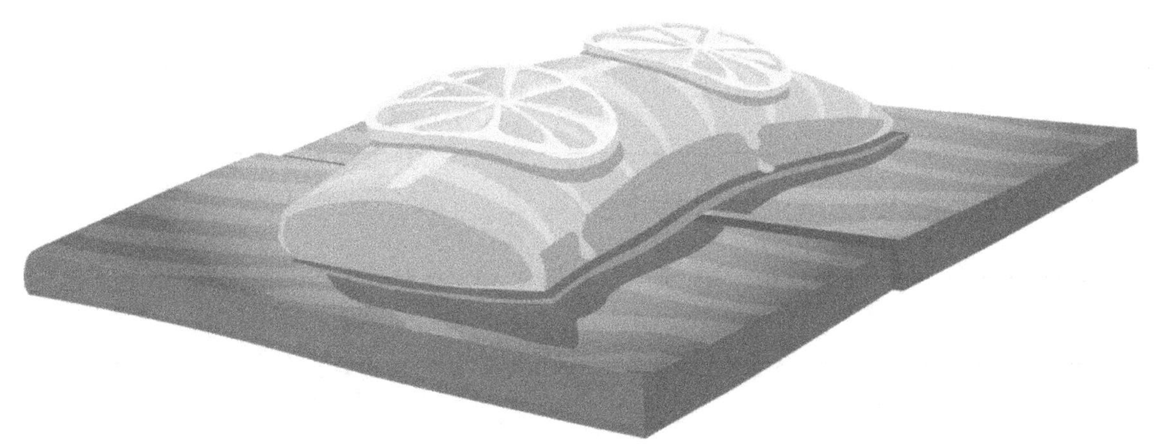

Meal Planner

Day 1	Breakfast: Lunch: Dinner:
Day 2	Breakfast: Lunch: Dinner:
Day 3	Breakfast: Lunch: Dinner:
Day 4	Breakfast: Lunch: Dinner:
Day 5	Breakfast: Lunch: Dinner:
Day 6	Breakfast: Lunch: Dinner:
Day 7	Breakfast: Lunch: Dinner:
Snacks	

Exercise Tracker

Day 50 - 56

Day 1	Day 2	Day 3
Cardio ○ Weights ○	Cardio ○ Weights ○	Cardio ○ Weights ○

Day 4	Day 5	Day 6
Cardio ○ Weights ○	Cardio ○ Weights ○	Cardio ○ Weights ○

Day 7
Cardio ○   Weights ○

Day	Calories Burned
1	
2	
3	
4	
5	
6	
7	

Day 50   Food Tracker

Date: _______________

MON TUE WED THU FRI SAT SUN

🎯 Daily Target						
Breakfast	Calories	Fat	Protein	Carbs	Fiber	Net Carbs
Total:						
Lunch	Calories	Fat	Protein	Carbs	Fiber	Net Carbs
Total:						
Dinner	Calories	Fat	Protein	Carbs	Fiber	Net Carbs
Total:						
Snacks	Calories	Fat	Protein	Carbs	Fiber	Net Carbs
Total:						
Daily Total						

Ketosis: Y/N   Intermittent Fasting: From _____am/pm - To_____am/pm

Day 51   Food Tracker

Date: _______________
MON TUE WED THU FRI SAT SUN

⊕ Daily Target						
Breakfast	Calories	Fat	Protein	Carbs	Fiber	Net Carbs
Total:						
Lunch	Calories	Fat	Protein	Carbs	Fiber	Net Carbs
Total:						
Dinner	Calories	Fat	Protein	Carbs	Fiber	Net Carbs
Total:						
Snacks	Calories	Fat	Protein	Carbs	Fiber	Net Carbs
Total:						
Daily Total						

Ketosis: Y/N   Intermittent Fasting: From _____am/pm - To_____am/pm

Day 52   Food Tracker

Date: _______________

MON TUE WED THU FRI SAT SUN

🎯 **Daily Target**						

Breakfast	Calories	Fat	Protein	Carbs	Fiber	Net Carbs
Total:						

Lunch	Calories	Fat	Protein	Carbs	Fiber	Net Carbs
Total:						

Dinner	Calories	Fat	Protein	Carbs	Fiber	Net Carbs
Total:						

Snacks	Calories	Fat	Protein	Carbs	Fiber	Net Carbs
Total:						

Daily Total						

Ketosis: Y/N   Intermittent Fasting: From _____am/pm - To_____am/pm

Day 53   Food Tracker

Date: ________________

MON TUE WED THU FRI SAT SUN

⊕ Daily Target						

Breakfast	Calories	Fat	Protein	Carbs	Fiber	Net Carbs
Total:						

Lunch	Calories	Fat	Protein	Carbs	Fiber	Net Carbs
Total:						

Dinner	Calories	Fat	Protein	Carbs	Fiber	Net Carbs
Total:						

Snacks	Calories	Fat	Protein	Carbs	Fiber	Net Carbs
Total:						

Daily Total						

Ketosis: Y/N   Intermittent Fasting: From _______am/pm - To_______am/pm

Day 54   Food Tracker

Date: __________________

MON TUE WED THU FRI SAT SUN

🎯 Daily Target						
Breakfast	Calories	Fat	Protein	Carbs	Fiber	Net Carbs
Total:						
Lunch	Calories	Fat	Protein	Carbs	Fiber	Net Carbs
Total:						
Dinner	Calories	Fat	Protein	Carbs	Fiber	Net Carbs
Total:						
Snacks	Calories	Fat	Protein	Carbs	Fiber	Net Carbs
Total:						
Daily Total						

Ketosis: Y/N   Intermittent Fasting: From ____am/pm - To____am/pm

Day 55   Food Tracker

Date: __________________

MON TUE WED THU FRI SAT SUN

⊕ **Daily Target**						

Breakfast	Calories	Fat	Protein	Carbs	Fiber	Net Carbs
Total:						

Lunch	Calories	Fat	Protein	Carbs	Fiber	Net Carbs
Total:						

Dinner	Calories	Fat	Protein	Carbs	Fiber	Net Carbs
Total:						

Snacks	Calories	Fat	Protein	Carbs	Fiber	Net Carbs
Total:						

Daily Total						

Ketosis: Y/N   Intermittent Fasting: From _____am/pm - To_____am/pm

Day 56   Food Tracker

Date: ______________
MON TUE WED THU FRI SAT SUN

⊕ **Daily Target**						

Breakfast	Calories	Fat	Protein	Carbs	Fiber	Net Carbs
Total:						

Lunch	Calories	Fat	Protein	Carbs	Fiber	Net Carbs
Total:						

Dinner	Calories	Fat	Protein	Carbs	Fiber	Net Carbs
Total:						

Snacks	Calories	Fat	Protein	Carbs	Fiber	Net Carbs
Total:						

Daily Total						

Ketosis: Y/N   Intermittent Fasting: From _____am/pm - To_____am/pm

NOTES

DAY 57 – WEIGHT

Measurements

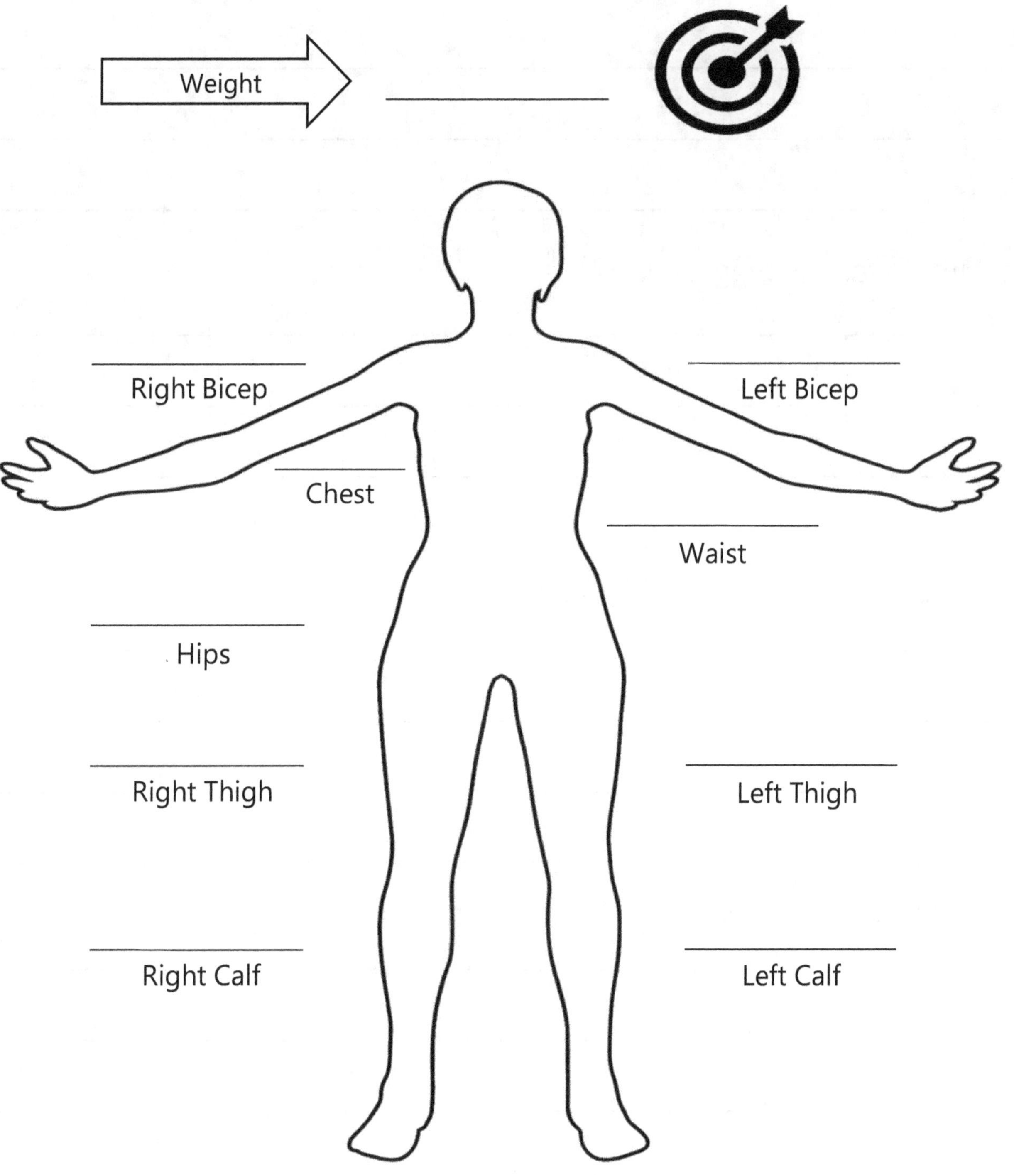

Questions To Ask Yourself

Am I happy with my results after the last 7 days?

What was my biggest win?

What adjustments should I make?

How does my body feel?

DAY 57 - 63

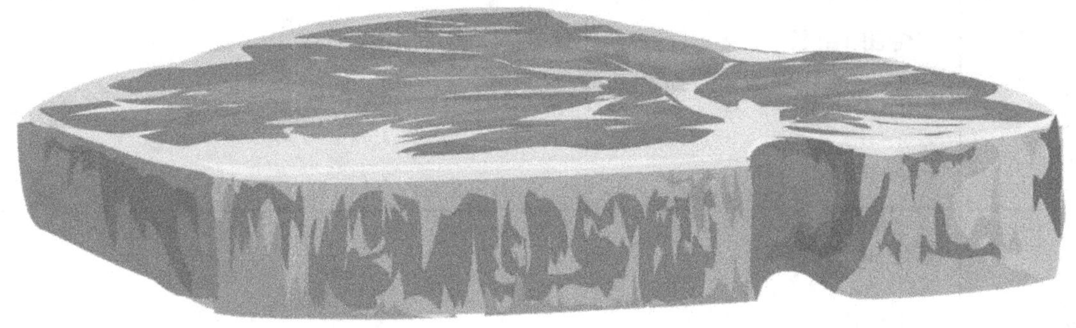

Meal Planner

Day 57 - 63

Day 1	Breakfast: Lunch: Dinner:
Day 2	Breakfast: Lunch: Dinner:
Day 3	Breakfast: Lunch: Dinner:
Day 4	Breakfast: Lunch: Dinner:
Day 5	Breakfast: Lunch: Dinner:
Day 6	Breakfast: Lunch: Dinner:
Day 7	Breakfast: Lunch: Dinner:
Snacks	

Exercise Tracker

Day 1	Day 2	Day 3
Cardio ○ Weights ○	Cardio ○ Weights ○	Cardio ○ Weights ○

Day 4	Day 5	Day 6
Cardio ○ Weights ○	Cardio ○ Weights ○	Cardio ○ Weights ○

Day 7
Cardio ○ Weights ○

Day	Calories Burned
1	
2	
3	
4	
5	
6	
7	

Day 57   Food Tracker

Date: ________________

MON TUE WED THU FRI SAT SUN

⊕ **Daily Target**						

Breakfast	Calories	Fat	Protein	Carbs	Fiber	Net Carbs
Total:						

Lunch	Calories	Fat	Protein	Carbs	Fiber	Net Carbs
Total:						

Dinner	Calories	Fat	Protein	Carbs	Fiber	Net Carbs
Total:						

Snacks	Calories	Fat	Protein	Carbs	Fiber	Net Carbs
Total:						

Daily Total						

Ketosis: Y/N   Intermittent Fasting: From _____am/pm - To_____am/pm

Day 58　　Food Tracker

Date: ___________
MON TUE WED THU FRI SAT SUN

⊕ Daily Target						

Breakfast	Calories	Fat	Protein	Carbs	Fiber	Net Carbs
Total:						

Lunch	Calories	Fat	Protein	Carbs	Fiber	Net Carbs
Total:						

Dinner	Calories	Fat	Protein	Carbs	Fiber	Net Carbs
Total:						

Snacks	Calories	Fat	Protein	Carbs	Fiber	Net Carbs
Total:						

Daily Total						

Ketosis:　Y/N　　Intermittent Fasting: From _____am/pm - To_____am/pm

Day 59   Food Tracker

Date: ___________

MON TUE WED THU FRI SAT SUN

🎯 **Daily Target**					

Breakfast	Calories	Fat	Protein	Carbs	Fiber	Net Carbs
Total:						

Lunch	Calories	Fat	Protein	Carbs	Fiber	Net Carbs
Total:						

Dinner	Calories	Fat	Protein	Carbs	Fiber	Net Carbs
Total:						

Snacks	Calories	Fat	Protein	Carbs	Fiber	Net Carbs
Total:						

Daily Total						

Ketosis: Y/N   Intermittent Fasting: From _____am/pm - To_____am/pm

Day 60   Food Tracker

Date: _______________

MON TUE WED THU FRI SAT SUN

⌖ **Daily Target**						
Breakfast	Calories	Fat	Protein	Carbs	Fiber	Net Carbs
Total:						
Lunch	Calories	Fat	Protein	Carbs	Fiber	Net Carbs
Total:						
Dinner	Calories	Fat	Protein	Carbs	Fiber	Net Carbs
Total:						
Snacks	Calories	Fat	Protein	Carbs	Fiber	Net Carbs
Total:						
Daily Total						

Ketosis: Y/N   Intermittent Fasting: From _____am/pm - To_____am/pm

Day 61 Food Tracker

Date: ________________________

MON TUE WED THU FRI SAT SUN

🎯 **Daily Target**						
Breakfast	Calories	Fat	Protein	Carbs	Fiber	Net Carbs
Total:						
Lunch	Calories	Fat	Protein	Carbs	Fiber	Net Carbs
Total:						
Dinner	Calories	Fat	Protein	Carbs	Fiber	Net Carbs
Total:						
Snacks	Calories	Fat	Protein	Carbs	Fiber	Net Carbs
Total:						
Daily Total						

Ketosis: Y/N   Intermittent Fasting: From _____am/pm - To_____am/pm

Day 62 Food Tracker

Date: _______________

MON TUE WED THU FRI SAT SUN

⌖ **Daily Target**						

Breakfast	Calories	Fat	Protein	Carbs	Fiber	Net Carbs
Total:						

Lunch	Calories	Fat	Protein	Carbs	Fiber	Net Carbs
Total:						

Dinner	Calories	Fat	Protein	Carbs	Fiber	Net Carbs
Total:						

Snacks	Calories	Fat	Protein	Carbs	Fiber	Net Carbs
Total:						

Daily Total						

Ketosis: Y/N   Intermittent Fasting: From _____am/pm - To_____am/pm

Day 63   Food Tracker

Date: _______________
MON TUE WED THU FRI SAT SUN

⊕ **Daily Target**

Breakfast	Calories	Fat	Protein	Carbs	Fiber	Net Carbs
Total:						

Lunch	Calories	Fat	Protein	Carbs	Fiber	Net Carbs
Total:						

Dinner	Calories	Fat	Protein	Carbs	Fiber	Net Carbs
Total:						

Snacks	Calories	Fat	Protein	Carbs	Fiber	Net Carbs
Total:						

Daily Total						

Ketosis: Y/N   Intermittent Fasting: From _____am/pm - To_____am/pm

NOTES

DAY 64 – WEIGHT

Measurements

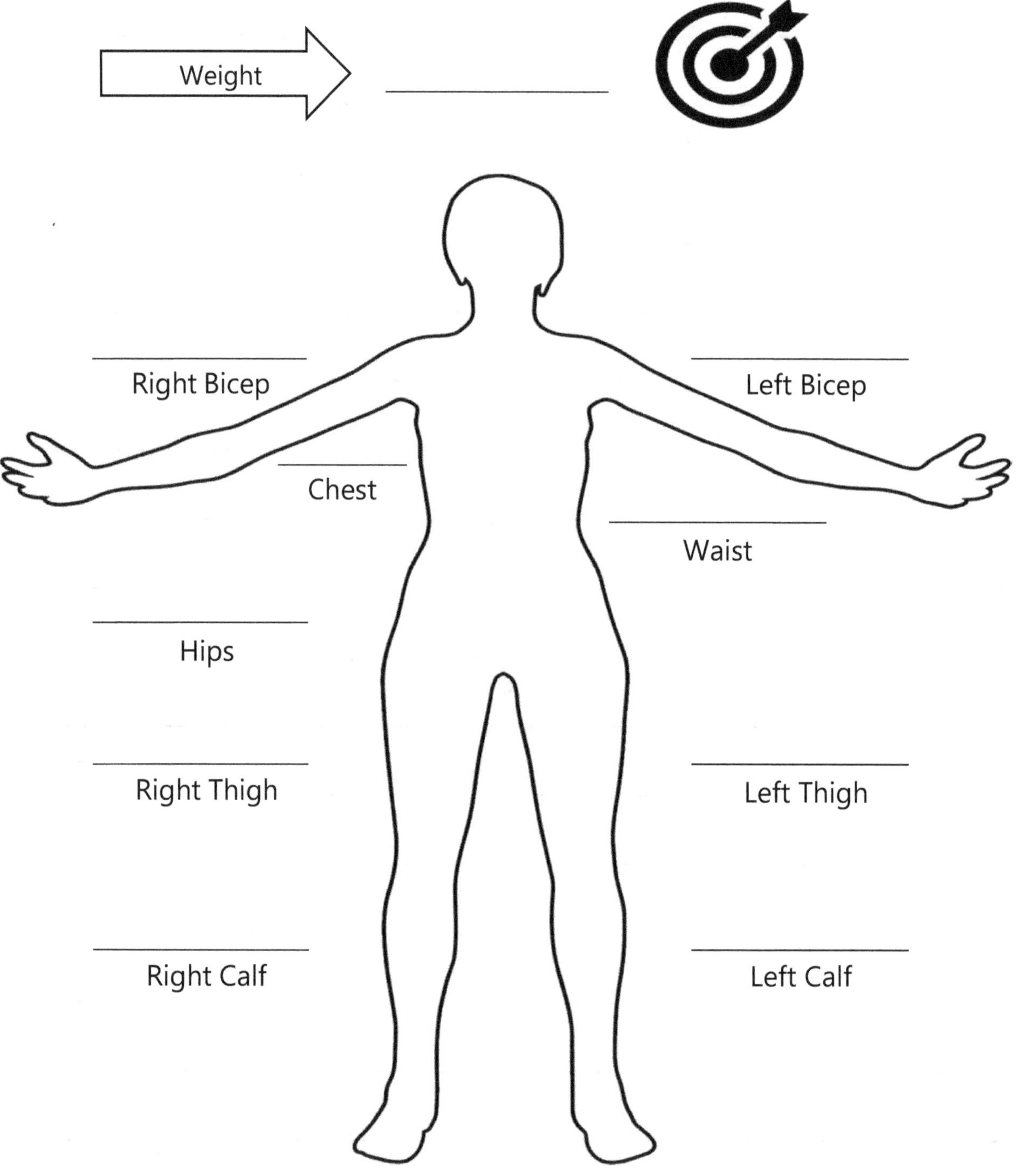

Questions To Ask Yourself

Am I happy with my results after the last 7 days?

____

____

____

____

What was my biggest win?

____

____

____

____

What adjustments should I make?

____

____

____

____

How does my body feel?

____

____

____

____

DAY 64 - 70

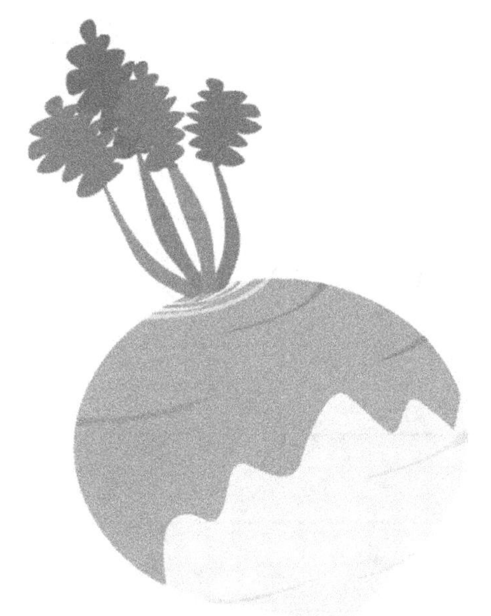

Meal Planner

Day 64 - 70

Day 1	Breakfast: Lunch: Dinner:
Day 2	Breakfast: Lunch: Dinner:
Day 3	Breakfast: Lunch: Dinner:
Day 4	Breakfast: Lunch: Dinner:
Day 5	Breakfast: Lunch: Dinner:
Day 6	Breakfast: Lunch: Dinner:
Day 7	Breakfast: Lunch: Dinner:
Snacks	

Exercise Tracker

Day 64 - 70

Day 1	Day 2	Day 3
Cardio ◯ Weights ◯	Cardio ◯ Weights ◯	Cardio ◯ Weights ◯
Day 4	Day 5	Day 6
Cardio ◯ Weights ◯	Cardio ◯ Weights ◯	Cardio ◯ Weights ◯

Day 7
Cardio ◯ Weights ◯

Day	Calories Burned
1	
2	
3	
4	
5	
6	
7	

Day 64   Food Tracker

Date: __________________

MON TUE WED THU FRI SAT SUN

⊕ Daily Target						

Breakfast	Calories	Fat	Protein	Carbs	Fiber	Net Carbs
Total:						

Lunch	Calories	Fat	Protein	Carbs	Fiber	Net Carbs
Total:						

Dinner	Calories	Fat	Protein	Carbs	Fiber	Net Carbs
Total:						

Snacks	Calories	Fat	Protein	Carbs	Fiber	Net Carbs
Total:						

Daily Total						

Ketosis: Y/N   Intermittent Fasting: From _____am/pm - To_____am/pm

Day 65   Food Tracker

Date: ________________

MON TUE WED THU FRI SAT SUN

⊕ **Daily Target**

Breakfast	Calories	Fat	Protein	Carbs	Fiber	Net Carbs
Total:						

Lunch	Calories	Fat	Protein	Carbs	Fiber	Net Carbs
Total:						

Dinner	Calories	Fat	Protein	Carbs	Fiber	Net Carbs
Total:						

Snacks	Calories	Fat	Protein	Carbs	Fiber	Net Carbs
Total:						

| **Daily Total** | | | | | | |

Ketosis: Y/N   Intermittent Fasting: From _____am/pm - To_____am/pm

Day 66   Food Tracker

Date: ________________

MON TUE WED THU FRI SAT SUN

🎯 Daily Target						

Breakfast	Calories	Fat	Protein	Carbs	Fiber	Net Carbs
Total:						

Lunch	Calories	Fat	Protein	Carbs	Fiber	Net Carbs
Total:						

Dinner	Calories	Fat	Protein	Carbs	Fiber	Net Carbs
Total:						

Snacks	Calories	Fat	Protein	Carbs	Fiber	Net Carbs
Total:						

Daily Total						

Ketosis: Y/N   Intermittent Fasting: From _____am/pm - To_____am/pm

Day 67   Food Tracker

Date: ________________

MON TUE WED THU FRI SAT SUN

🎯 Daily Target						

Breakfast	Calories	Fat	Protein	Carbs	Fiber	Net Carbs
Total:						

Lunch	Calories	Fat	Protein	Carbs	Fiber	Net Carbs
Total:						

Dinner	Calories	Fat	Protein	Carbs	Fiber	Net Carbs
Total:						

Snacks	Calories	Fat	Protein	Carbs	Fiber	Net Carbs
Total:						

Daily Total						

Ketosis: Y/N   Intermittent Fasting: From ______am/pm - To______am/pm

Day 68   Food Tracker

Date: _______________

MON TUE WED THU FRI SAT SUN

⊕ Daily Target						

Breakfast	Calories	Fat	Protein	Carbs	Fiber	Net Carbs
Total:						

Lunch	Calories	Fat	Protein	Carbs	Fiber	Net Carbs
Total:						

Dinner	Calories	Fat	Protein	Carbs	Fiber	Net Carbs
Total:						

Snacks	Calories	Fat	Protein	Carbs	Fiber	Net Carbs
Total:						

Daily Total						

Ketosis: Y/N   Intermittent Fasting: From _____am/pm - To_____am/pm

Day 69　　Food Tracker

Date: ________________
MON TUE WED THU FRI SAT SUN

🎯 **Daily Target**						

Breakfast	Calories	Fat	Protein	Carbs	Fiber	Net Carbs
Total:						

Lunch	Calories	Fat	Protein	Carbs	Fiber	Net Carbs
Total:						

Dinner	Calories	Fat	Protein	Carbs	Fiber	Net Carbs
Total:						

Snacks	Calories	Fat	Protein	Carbs	Fiber	Net Carbs
Total:						

Daily Total						

Ketosis:　Y/N　　Intermittent Fasting: From ______am/pm - To______am/pm

Day 70   Food Tracker

Date: ________________

MON TUE WED THU FRI SAT SUN

⌖ Daily Target						

Breakfast	Calories	Fat	Protein	Carbs	Fiber	Net Carbs
Total:						

Lunch	Calories	Fat	Protein	Carbs	Fiber	Net Carbs
Total:						

Dinner	Calories	Fat	Protein	Carbs	Fiber	Net Carbs
Total:						

Snacks	Calories	Fat	Protein	Carbs	Fiber	Net Carbs
Total:						

Daily Total						

Ketosis: Y/N   Intermittent Fasting: From ____am/pm - To____am/pm

NOTES

DAY 71 – WEIGHT

Measurements

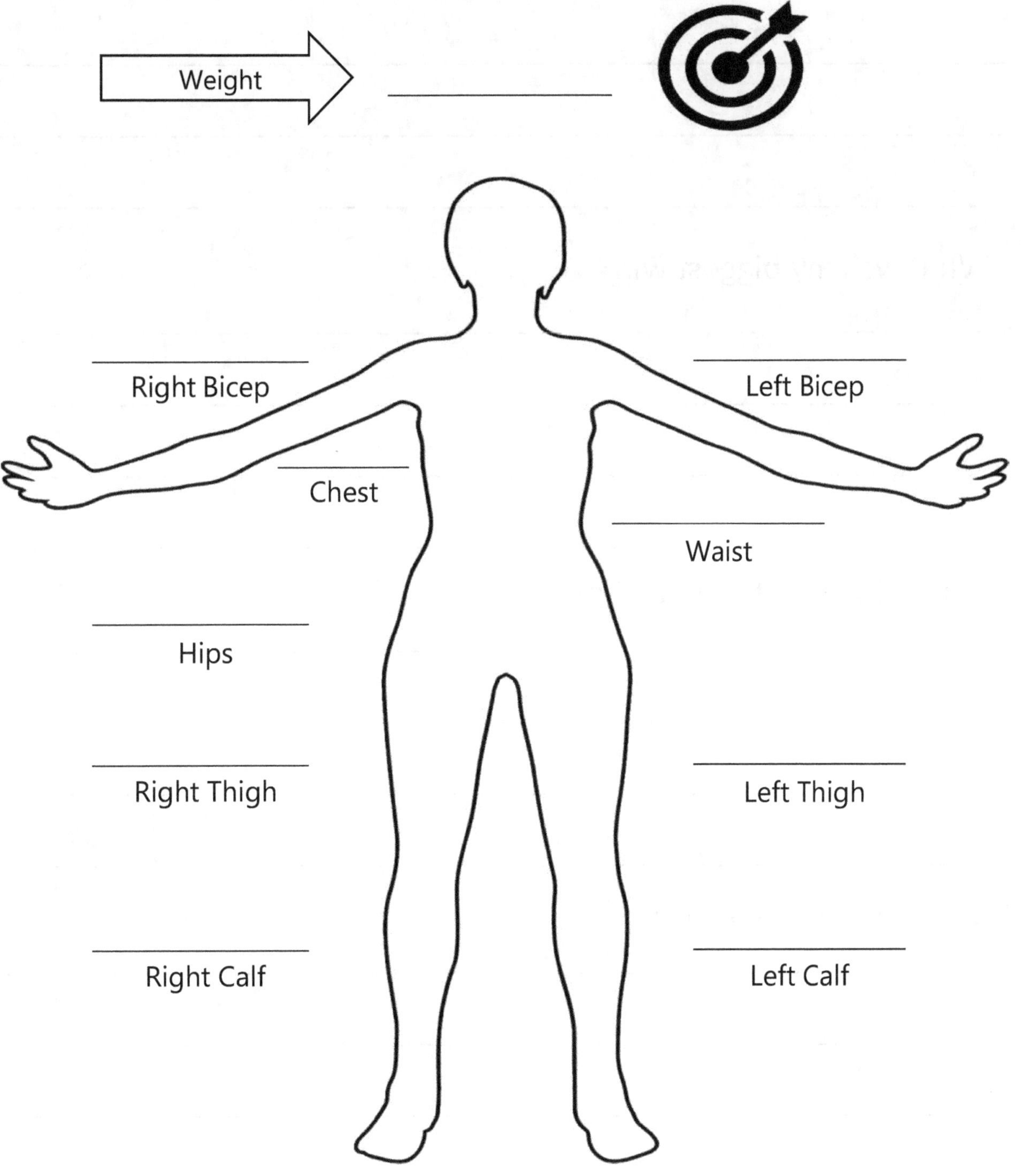

Questions To Ask Yourself

Am I happy with my results after the last 7 days?

____

____

____

What was my biggest win?

____

____

____

What adjustments should I make?

____

____

____

How does my body feel?

____

____

____

DAY 71 - 77

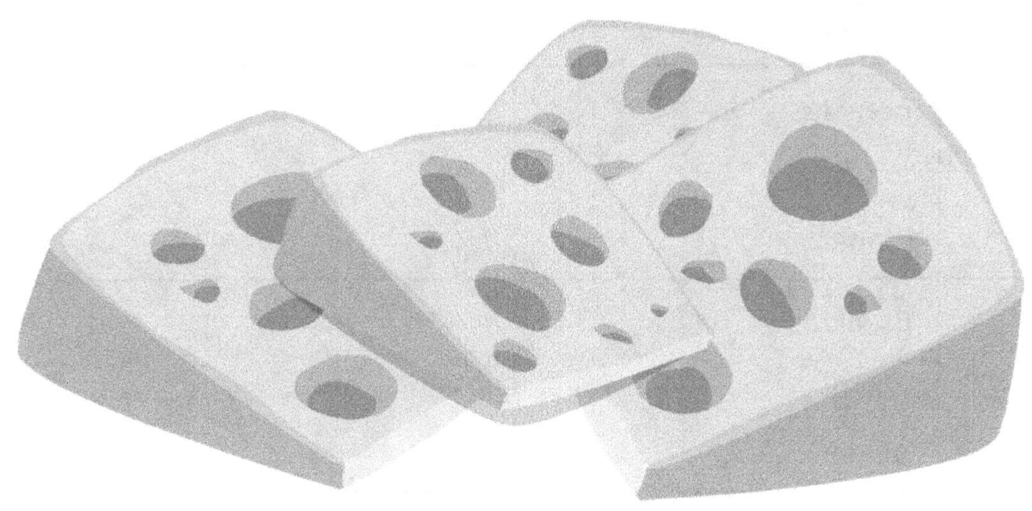

Meal Planner

Day 1	Breakfast: Lunch: Dinner:
Day 2	Breakfast: Lunch: Dinner:
Day 3	Breakfast: Lunch: Dinner:
Day 4	Breakfast: Lunch: Dinner:
Day 5	Breakfast: Lunch: Dinner:
Day 6	Breakfast: Lunch: Dinner:
Day 7	Breakfast: Lunch: Dinner:
Snacks	

Exercise Tracker

Day 71 - 77

Day 1	Day 2	Day 3
Cardio ◯ Weights ◯	Cardio ◯ Weights ◯	Cardio ◯ Weights ◯

Day 4	Day 5	Day 6
Cardio ◯ Weights ◯	Cardio ◯ Weights ◯	Cardio ◯ Weights ◯

Day 7
Cardio ◯ Weights ◯

Day	Calories Burned
1	
2	
3	
4	
5	
6	
7	

Day 71   Food Tracker

Date: ________________
MON TUE WED THU FRI SAT SUN

⊕ Daily Target						

Breakfast	Calories	Fat	Protein	Carbs	Fiber	Net Carbs
Total:						

Lunch	Calories	Fat	Protein	Carbs	Fiber	Net Carbs
Total:						

Dinner	Calories	Fat	Protein	Carbs	Fiber	Net Carbs
Total:						

Snacks	Calories	Fat	Protein	Carbs	Fiber	Net Carbs
Total:						

Daily Total						

Ketosis: Y/N   Intermittent Fasting: From _____am/pm - To_____am/pm

Day 72   Food Tracker

Date: ______________________
MON TUE WED THU FRI SAT SUN

⊕ **Daily Target**						
Breakfast	Calories	Fat	Protein	Carbs	Fiber	Net Carbs
Total:						
Lunch	Calories	Fat	Protein	Carbs	Fiber	Net Carbs
Total:						
Dinner	Calories	Fat	Protein	Carbs	Fiber	Net Carbs
Total:						
Snacks	Calories	Fat	Protein	Carbs	Fiber	Net Carbs
Total:						
Daily Total						

Ketosis: Y/N   Intermittent Fasting: From _____am/pm - To_____am/pm

Day 73   Food Tracker

Date: ___________________

MON TUE WED THU FRI SAT SUN

⊕ **Daily Target**						

Breakfast	Calories	Fat	Protein	Carbs	Fiber	Net Carbs
Total:						

Lunch	Calories	Fat	Protein	Carbs	Fiber	Net Carbs
Total:						

Dinner	Calories	Fat	Protein	Carbs	Fiber	Net Carbs
Total:						

Snacks	Calories	Fat	Protein	Carbs	Fiber	Net Carbs
Total:						

Daily Total						

Ketosis: Y/N   Intermittent Fasting: From _____am/pm - To_____am/pm

Day 74 Food Tracker

Date: ________________

MON TUE WED THU FRI SAT SUN

⊕ **Daily Target**

Breakfast	Calories	Fat	Protein	Carbs	Fiber	Net Carbs
Total:						

Lunch	Calories	Fat	Protein	Carbs	Fiber	Net Carbs
Total:						

Dinner	Calories	Fat	Protein	Carbs	Fiber	Net Carbs
Total:						

Snacks	Calories	Fat	Protein	Carbs	Fiber	Net Carbs
Total:						

| **Daily Total** | | | | | | |

Ketosis: Y/N   Intermittent Fasting: From _____am/pm - To_____am/pm

Day 75   Food Tracker

Date: ________________
MON TUE WED THU FRI SAT SUN

🎯 **Daily Target**						

Breakfast	Calories	Fat	Protein	Carbs	Fiber	Net Carbs
Total:						

Lunch	Calories	Fat	Protein	Carbs	Fiber	Net Carbs
Total:						

Dinner	Calories	Fat	Protein	Carbs	Fiber	Net Carbs
Total:						

Snacks	Calories	Fat	Protein	Carbs	Fiber	Net Carbs
Total:						

Daily Total						

Ketosis: Y/N   Intermittent Fasting: From _____am/pm - To_____am/pm

Day 76   Food Tracker

Date: ________________

MON TUE WED THU FRI SAT SUN

🎯 Daily Target						

Breakfast	Calories	Fat	Protein	Carbs	Fiber	Net Carbs
Total:						

Lunch	Calories	Fat	Protein	Carbs	Fiber	Net Carbs
Total:						

Dinner	Calories	Fat	Protein	Carbs	Fiber	Net Carbs
Total:						

Snacks	Calories	Fat	Protein	Carbs	Fiber	Net Carbs
Total:						

Daily Total						

Ketosis: Y/N   Intermittent Fasting: From _____am/pm - To_____am/pm

Day 77   Food Tracker

Date: ______________

MON TUE WED THU FRI SAT SUN

⊕ Daily Target						

Breakfast	Calories	Fat	Protein	Carbs	Fiber	Net Carbs
Total:						

Lunch	Calories	Fat	Protein	Carbs	Fiber	Net Carbs
Total:						

Dinner	Calories	Fat	Protein	Carbs	Fiber	Net Carbs
Total:						

Snacks	Calories	Fat	Protein	Carbs	Fiber	Net Carbs
Total:						

Daily Total						

Ketosis: Y/N   Intermittent Fasting: From _____am/pm - To_____am/pm

NOTES

DAY 78 – WEIGHT

Measurements

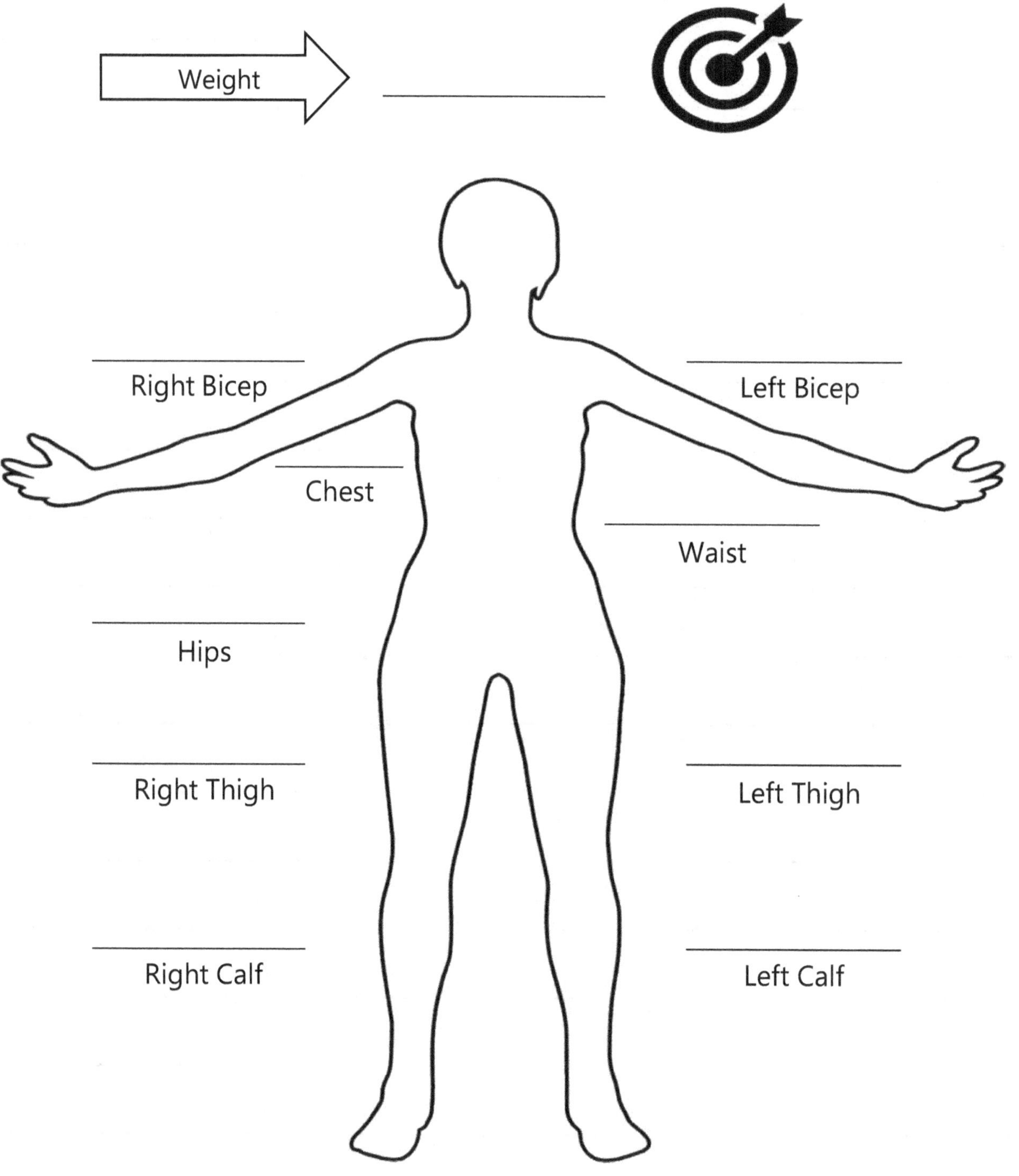

Questions To Ask Yourself

Am I happy with my results after the last 7 days?

____

____

____

____

What was my biggest win?

____

____

____

____

What adjustments should I make?

____

____

____

____

How does my body feel?

____

____

____

____

DAY 78 - 84

Meal Planner

Day 78 - 84

Day 1	Breakfast: Lunch: Dinner:
Day 2	Breakfast: Lunch: Dinner:
Day 3	Breakfast: Lunch: Dinner:
Day 4	Breakfast: Lunch: Dinner:
Day 5	Breakfast: Lunch: Dinner:
Day 6	Breakfast: Lunch: Dinner:
Day 7	Breakfast: Lunch: Dinner:
Snacks	

Exercise Tracker   Day 78 - 84

Day 1

Cardio ○
Weights ○

Day 2

Cardio ○
Weights ○

Day 3

Cardio ○
Weights ○

Day 4

Cardio ○
Weights ○

Day 5

Cardio ○
Weights ○

Day 6

Cardio ○
Weights ○

Day 7

Cardio ○
Weights ○

Day	Calories Burned
1	
2	
3	
4	
5	
6	
7	

Day 78   Food Tracker

Date: _______________

MON TUE WED THU FRI SAT SUN

⊕ **Daily Target**						
Breakfast	Calories	Fat	Protein	Carbs	Fiber	Net Carbs
Total:						
Lunch	Calories	Fat	Protein	Carbs	Fiber	Net Carbs
Total:						
Dinner	Calories	Fat	Protein	Carbs	Fiber	Net Carbs
Total:						
Snacks	Calories	Fat	Protein	Carbs	Fiber	Net Carbs
Total:						
Daily Total						

Ketosis: Y/N   Intermittent Fasting: From _____am/pm - To_____am/pm

Day 79   Food Tracker

Date: ______________________

MON TUE WED THU FRI SAT SUN

⊕ Daily Target						

Breakfast	Calories	Fat	Protein	Carbs	Fiber	Net Carbs
Total:						

Lunch	Calories	Fat	Protein	Carbs	Fiber	Net Carbs
Total:						

Dinner	Calories	Fat	Protein	Carbs	Fiber	Net Carbs
Total:						

Snacks	Calories	Fat	Protein	Carbs	Fiber	Net Carbs
Total:						

Daily Total						

Ketosis: Y/N   Intermittent Fasting: From ______am/pm - To______am/pm

Day 80   Food Tracker

Date: ______________
MON TUE WED THU FRI SAT SUN

⊕ **Daily Target**

Breakfast	Calories	Fat	Protein	Carbs	Fiber	Net Carbs
Total:						

Lunch	Calories	Fat	Protein	Carbs	Fiber	Net Carbs
Total:						

Dinner	Calories	Fat	Protein	Carbs	Fiber	Net Carbs
Total:						

Snacks	Calories	Fat	Protein	Carbs	Fiber	Net Carbs
Total:						

| **Daily Total** | | | | | | |

Ketosis: Y/N   Intermittent Fasting: From _____am/pm - To_____am/pm

Day 81   Food Tracker

Date: _______________

MON TUE WED THU FRI SAT SUN

⊕ **Daily Target**

Breakfast	Calories	Fat	Protein	Carbs	Fiber	Net Carbs
Total:						

Lunch	Calories	Fat	Protein	Carbs	Fiber	Net Carbs
Total:						

Dinner	Calories	Fat	Protein	Carbs	Fiber	Net Carbs
Total:						

Snacks	Calories	Fat	Protein	Carbs	Fiber	Net Carbs
Total:						

| **Daily Total** | | | | | | |

Ketosis: Y/N   Intermittent Fasting: From _____am/pm - To_____am/pm

Day 82   Food Tracker

Date: ________________
MON TUE WED THU FRI SAT SUN

⊕ **Daily Target**

Breakfast	Calories	Fat	Protein	Carbs	Fiber	Net Carbs
Total:						

Lunch	Calories	Fat	Protein	Carbs	Fiber	Net Carbs
Total:						

Dinner	Calories	Fat	Protein	Carbs	Fiber	Net Carbs
Total:						

Snacks	Calories	Fat	Protein	Carbs	Fiber	Net Carbs
Total:						

| **Daily Total** | | | | | | |

Ketosis: Y/N   Intermittent Fasting: From _____am/pm - To_____am/pm

Day 83   Food Tracker

Date: ___________

MON TUE WED THU FRI SAT SUN

🎯 **Daily Target**

Breakfast	Calories	Fat	Protein	Carbs	Fiber	Net Carbs
Total:						

Lunch	Calories	Fat	Protein	Carbs	Fiber	Net Carbs
Total:						

Dinner	Calories	Fat	Protein	Carbs	Fiber	Net Carbs
Total:						

Snacks	Calories	Fat	Protein	Carbs	Fiber	Net Carbs
Total:						
Daily Total						

Ketosis: Y/N   Intermittent Fasting: From ____am/pm - To____am/pm

Day 84   Food Tracker

Date: _______________

MON TUE WED THU FRI SAT SUN

⊕ **Daily Target**						

Breakfast	Calories	Fat	Protein	Carbs	Fiber	Net Carbs
Total:						

Lunch	Calories	Fat	Protein	Carbs	Fiber	Net Carbs
Total:						

Dinner	Calories	Fat	Protein	Carbs	Fiber	Net Carbs
Total:						

Snacks	Calories	Fat	Protein	Carbs	Fiber	Net Carbs
Total:						

Daily Total						

Ketosis: Y/N   Intermittent Fasting: From _____am/pm - To_____am/pm

NOTES

DAY 85 – WEIGHT

Measurements

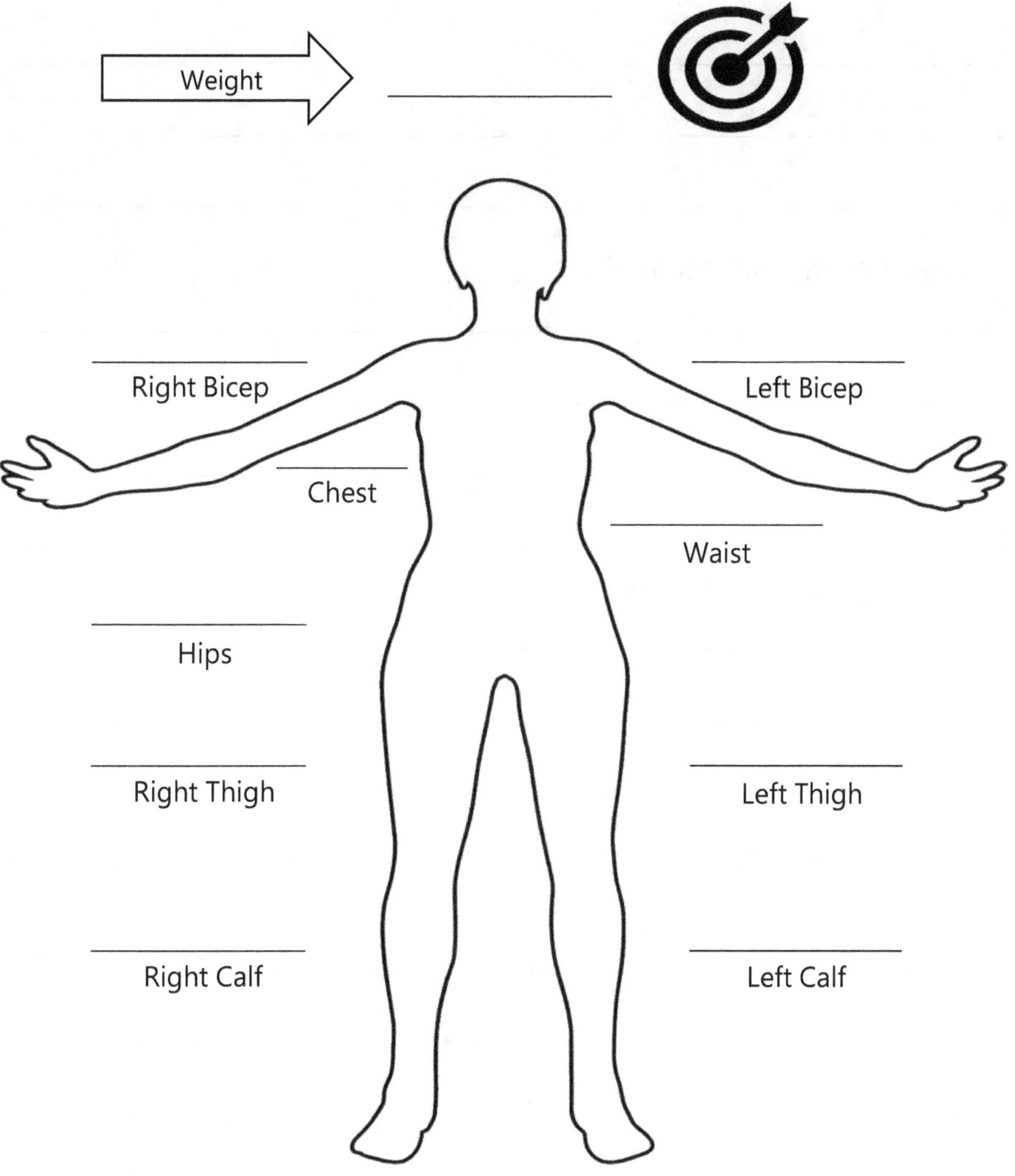

Questions To Ask Yourself

Am I happy with my results after the last 7 days?

What was my biggest win?

What adjustments should I make?

How does my body feel?

DAY 85 - 90

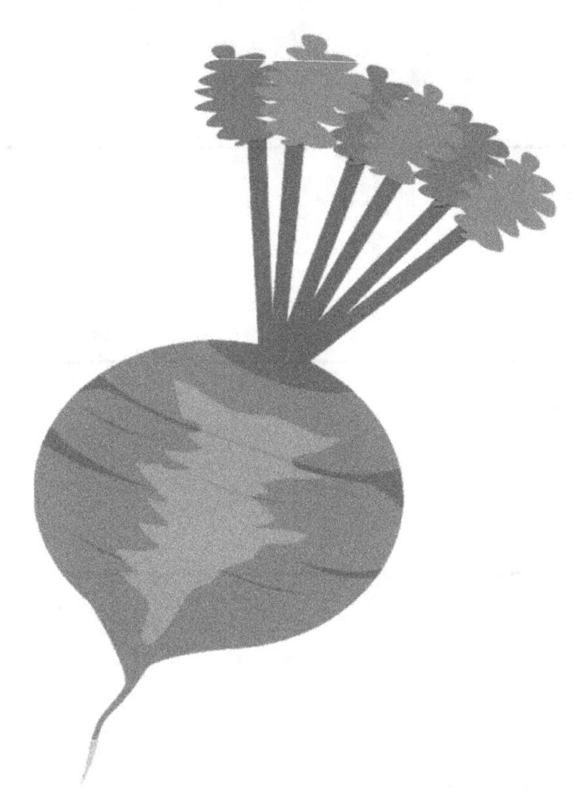

Meal Planner Day 85 - 90

Day 1	Breakfast: Lunch: Dinner:
Day 2	Breakfast: Lunch: Dinner:
Day 3	Breakfast: Lunch: Dinner:
Day 4	Breakfast: Lunch: Dinner:
Day 5	Breakfast: Lunch: Dinner:
Day 6	Breakfast: Lunch: Dinner:
Day 7	Breakfast: Lunch: Dinner:
Snacks	

Exercise Tracker Day 85 - 90

Day 1
Cardio ◯   Weights ◯

Day 2
Cardio ◯   Weights ◯

Day 3
Cardio ◯   Weights ◯

Day 4
Cardio ◯   Weights ◯

Day 5
Cardio ◯   Weights ◯

Day 6
Cardio ◯   Weights ◯

Day 7
Cardio ◯   Weights ◯

Day	Calories Burned
1	
2	
3	
4	
5	
6	
7	

Day 85   Food Tracker

Date: _______________________

MON TUE WED THU FRI SAT SUN

🎯 Daily Target						

Breakfast	Calories	Fat	Protein	Carbs	Fiber	Net Carbs
Total:						

Lunch	Calories	Fat	Protein	Carbs	Fiber	Net Carbs
Total:						

Dinner	Calories	Fat	Protein	Carbs	Fiber	Net Carbs
Total:						

Snacks	Calories	Fat	Protein	Carbs	Fiber	Net Carbs
Total:						

Daily Total						

Ketosis: Y/N   Intermittent Fasting: From ____am/pm - To____am/pm

Day 86   Food Tracker

Date: _______________

MON TUE WED THU FRI SAT SUN

⊕ **Daily Target**

Breakfast	Calories	Fat	Protein	Carbs	Fiber	Net Carbs
Total:						

Lunch	Calories	Fat	Protein	Carbs	Fiber	Net Carbs
Total:						

Dinner	Calories	Fat	Protein	Carbs	Fiber	Net Carbs
Total:						

Snacks	Calories	Fat	Protein	Carbs	Fiber	Net Carbs
Total:						

| **Daily Total** | | | | | | |

Ketosis: Y/N   Intermittent Fasting: From _____am/pm - To_____am/pm

Day 87 — Food Tracker

Date: _______________

MON TUE WED THU FRI SAT SUN

🎯 **Daily Target**						

Breakfast	Calories	Fat	Protein	Carbs	Fiber	Net Carbs
Total:						

Lunch	Calories	Fat	Protein	Carbs	Fiber	Net Carbs
Total:						

Dinner	Calories	Fat	Protein	Carbs	Fiber	Net Carbs
Total:						

Snacks	Calories	Fat	Protein	Carbs	Fiber	Net Carbs
Total:						

Daily Total						

Ketosis: Y/N   Intermittent Fasting: From _______am/pm - To_______am/pm

Day 88 Food Tracker

Date: ________________

MON TUE WED THU FRI SAT SUN

⌖ Daily Target						

Breakfast	Calories	Fat	Protein	Carbs	Fiber	Net Carbs
Total:						

Lunch	Calories	Fat	Protein	Carbs	Fiber	Net Carbs
Total:						

Dinner	Calories	Fat	Protein	Carbs	Fiber	Net Carbs
Total:						

Snacks	Calories	Fat	Protein	Carbs	Fiber	Net Carbs
Total:						

Daily Total						

Ketosis: Y/N   Intermittent Fasting: From _____am/pm - To_____am/pm

Day 89　Food Tracker

Date: ___________________

MON TUE WED THU FRI SAT SUN

⊙ **Daily Target**					

Breakfast	Calories	Fat	Protein	Carbs	Fiber	Net Carbs
Total:						

Lunch	Calories	Fat	Protein	Carbs	Fiber	Net Carbs
Total:						

Dinner	Calories	Fat	Protein	Carbs	Fiber	Net Carbs
Total:						

Snacks	Calories	Fat	Protein	Carbs	Fiber	Net Carbs
Total:						

Daily Total					

Ketosis: Y/N　　Intermittent Fasting: From _____am/pm - To_____am/pm

Day 90   Food Tracker

Date: _______________

MON TUE WED THU FRI SAT SUN

◎ **Daily Target**

Breakfast	Calories	Fat	Protein	Carbs	Fiber	Net Carbs
Total:						

Lunch	Calories	Fat	Protein	Carbs	Fiber	Net Carbs
Total:						

Dinner	Calories	Fat	Protein	Carbs	Fiber	Net Carbs
Total:						

Snacks	Calories	Fat	Protein	Carbs	Fiber	Net Carbs
Total:						
Daily Total						

Ketosis: Y/N   Intermittent Fasting: From _____am/pm - To_____am/pm

NOTES

DAY 90 – ENDING WEIGHT

Measurements

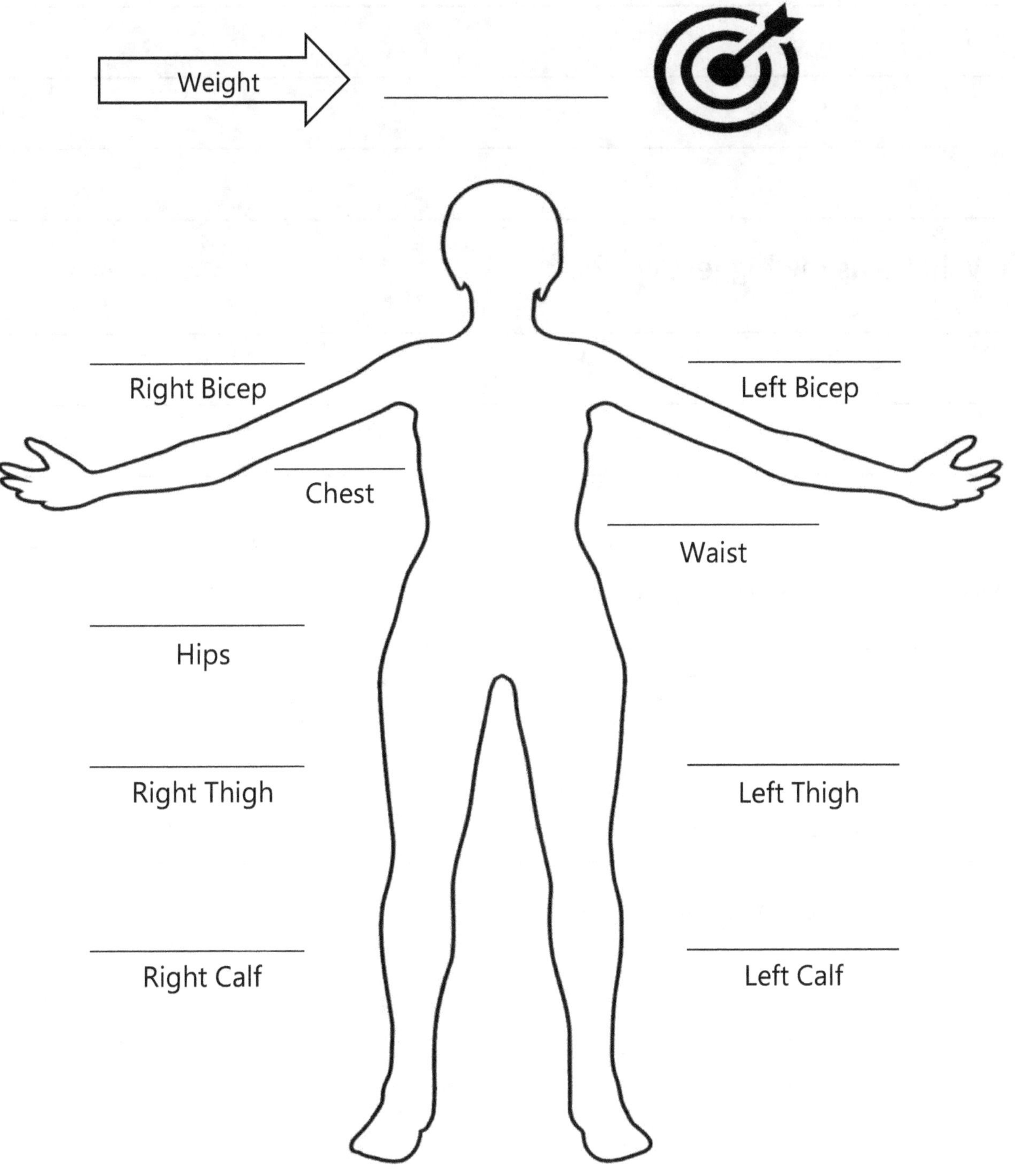

Questions To Ask Yourself

Am I happy with my results after the last 90 days?

____

____

____

What was my biggest win?

____

____

____

What adjustments should I make?

____

____

____

How does my body feel?

____

____

____

NOTES

NOTES

NOTES

NOTES

NOTES